AF790706

Genetics of Bipolar Disorder

Susanne Bengesser / Eva Reininghaus

Genetics of Bipolar Disorder

PL ACADEMIC RESEARCH

Bibliographic Information published by the Deutsche Nationalbibliothek
The Deutsche Nationalbibliothek lists this publication in the Deutsche Nationalbibliografie; detailed bibliographic data is available in the internet at http://dnb.d-nb.de.

Cover Illustration:
© Susanne Bengesser

Library of Congress Cataloging-in-Publication Data

Bengesser, Susanne, 1983-
Genetics of bipolar disorder / Susanne Bengesser, Eva Reininghaus.
p. ; cm.
Includes bibliographical references.
ISBN 978-3-631-63572-8
I. Reininghaus, Eva. II. Title.
[DNLM: 1. Bipolar Disorder—genetics. 2. Bipolar Disorder—therapy.
3. Genetic Predisposition to Disease. WM 207]
RC516
616.89'5—dc23
2013011915

ISBN 978-3-631-63572-8

© Peter Lang GmbH
Internationaler Verlag der Wissenschaften
Frankfurt am Main 2013
All rights reserved.
PL Academic Research is an Imprint of Peter Lang GmbH.

Peter Lang – Frankfurt am Main · Berlin · Bruxelles · New York · Oxford · Warszawa · Wien

All parts of this publication are protected by copyright. Any utilisation outside the strict limits of the copyright law, without the permission of the publisher, is forbidden and liable to prosecution. This applies in particular to reproductions, translations, microfilming, and storage and processing in electronic retrieval systems.

www.peterlang.de

Preface

This book „Genetics of Bipolar Disorder"originated from a very detailed thesis written by Susanne Bengesser under supervision of Eva Reininghaus and myself. Eva Reininghaus received the doctorate of Medicine in 2004 and the doctorate of Medical Science in 2008. Furthermore she did her training as assistant doctor for Psychiatry at the Medical University of Graz/ Department of Psychiatry. Since 2011 she has managed the research group for Bipolar Disorder at the University Hospital of Graz. Furthermore she has been a member of the "ConLiGen-Consortium" since 2012. Beside she performed a research period in Toronto/Canada in 2011. Susanne Bengesser studied Medicine and Molecular Biology (Bachelor degree) at the Medical University of Graz and the Karl-Franzens University of Graz (October 2002-April 2010). Then she spent a short research period in Ulm/Germany at the laboratory of the Anatomy department (iPS group) to gain experience in laboratory techniques. Furthermore she started to work as an assistant doctor for Psychiatry in Rankweil/Austria (1st of January 2011 until 30th of September 2011) and continued the training in Internal Medicine at the hospital "Elisabethinen" in Linz (1st of Oktober 2011 until 31st of March 2012). Finally she has started to work at the Medical University of Graz/ Department of Psychiatry on the 1st of April 2012. Since April she has worked in the outpatient department for Bipolar Disorder and the Bipolar Disorder research group managed by Eva Reininghaus. Finally the extension and update of the thesis resulted in this very detailed and exciting book about the genetic blueprint of Bipolar Disorder, which pictures the complex current knowledge of science in a clear and understandable way. A chapter about the basic principles of genetics enables also reader with minor (or even without) genetic knowledge to deepen with the complex issue. Altogether this is a successful and professional summary of the genetics of Bipolar Disorder.

Graz, 30th of January — Prof. DDr. Hans-Peter Kapfhammer

Abstract

Bipolar disorder is a highly heritable disease with a polygenetic mode of inheritance. Although molecular psychiatry is still in its infancy, a huge amount of possible susceptibility genes have been discovered, but still with inconsistent results. Top susceptibility genes belong to channelopathies and ion channel associated proteins; especially ANK3 and CACNA1C are important susceptibility genes. A gene coding for the brain derived neurotrophic factor, BDNF, seems to be associated with bipolar disorder in Caucasians, but not in Asians. It could be a laboratory marker for bipolar disorder, because serum levels are decreased in patients with bipolar disorder. Another promising predisposing gene group includes the "clock genes", among which are ARNTL, CRY1, CRY2 and PER1-3. Although the serotonergic system might be expected to play a major role, because the neurotransmitter imbalance theory has dominated the pathogenesis of affective disorders for decades, serotonin receptor genes are not very likely to influence bipolar disorder to a major degree. The very well examined serotonin transporter polymorphisms are more likely to be involved in pathogenesis of manic-depressive disease. Other neurotransmitter systems, such as the dopamine and noradrenaline systems do not show overwhelming results either. The genes of the GABA and glutamate systems show some positive results. Beside those well-examined gene groups numerous newly detected possible susceptibility genes exist. A detailed description of all candidate genes and their polymorphisms is given within this book.The detection of all these susceptibility genes has great impact on future nosology and therapy. Boundaries between bipolar disorder and related diseases, for instance unipolar depression and schizophrenia, are blurred. Many possible susceptibility genes for bipolar disorder overlap with top candidates for schizophrenia, including CACNA1C, DISC1, COMT, DTNBP1, NRG1, DAOA and more. Bipolar disorder overlaps with major depression as well. Especially gene-variants of the serotonergic system, for example the well studied insertion/deletion serotonin transporter polymorphism, are shared between both affective disorders. Molecular psychiatry definitely will influence therapy decisions. Many genotypes of certain susceptibility genes lead to a better or worse response in pharmacological treatment. The short allele of the serotonin transporter promoter polymorphism leads for example to bad antidepressant response.

Genotypes have also an impact on the reaction toward environmental influences. While for instance some gene polymorphism milden the effects of childhood maltreatment, other gene variants aggravate depressive reaction after negative life events. All gene-environment-interactions and their implications for clinical practice are explained in depth in this review.

Acknowledgements

We would like to give special thanks to Nicole Spreitz for proofreading and editing.

Furthermore we want to thank Gerhard Bengesser for his special support.

This work was done using the facilities of the Medical University of Graz – we appreciate this possibility.

Table of Contents

1. Introduction

Many psychiatric diseases run within families and kinship. A high hereditary factor of mental disease was proven early through numerous family, twin and adoption studies. Important mental diseases such as Schizophrenia, Depression, Addiction, Autism, and Chorea Huntington have a strong genetic predisposition. With the exception of Chorea Huntington, those mental diseases do not show monogenetic pathogenesis, but a polygenetic inheritance. An orchestra of multiple, potentially interacting genes with small effects and incomplete penetrance lead to predisposition. Numerous possible susceptibility genes for psychiatric diseases are still unidentified and it is not exactly known how they interact to lead to illness.

Although molecular psychiatry is still in its infancy it is possible that in the future psychiatric genetics might help to draw exact lines between psychiatric diagnoses, which may lead to restructuring of nosology [Burmeister et al. 2008]. Furthermore, molecular genetics give insight in pathogenetic mechanisms, which will help to find targets for development of new medication and laboratory markers. Additionally, the knowledge of inheritance could lead to potent prevention strategies. However, one has to illuminate the gene-environment-interactions to detect plans against disease onset. Though molecular psychiatry still has to overcome initial difficulties, it is an attempt to review the genetics of bipolar affective disorder [Craddock et al. 2005].

1.1 Bipolar Affective Disorder

1.1.1 History and Symptomatology of Bipolar Disorder

Over centuries psychiatric terminology was confusing. Among the first to provide potential concepts were Araeteus from Cappadocia (50-130 A.D.), Jean Pierre Falret (1794-1870) and Jules Baillarges (1809 –1890). Over a century the essence of manic-depressive insanity was typically explained in Falret's term "folie circulaire" and Bailarger's "folie a double forme" [Benazzi et al. 2006; Haustgen et al. 2006]. However, their concepts were not sufficiently defined and not discerned enough [Alexander and Selesnick 1969; Angst et al. 2001]. Emil Kraepelin was the first to successfully coin the terms. He introduced the dualism of schizophrenia ("dementia praecox") and bipolar disorder ("manic depressive insanity") in a clear way. He described bipolar disorder as "manic depressive insanity" [Jablensky et al. 1999; Hippius et al. 2008]. Bipolar disorder is a mood disorder which includes depressive and manic episodes. Manic episodes are characterized by either elevated or dysphoric mood or a raised energy level. Other typical symptoms of mania are delusion of grandeur, logorrhea, racing thoughts, loss of social inhibitions, reduced requirement of sleep, hyper-sexuality, increased goal-directed activity or agitation, impulsive or high-risk behaviors for instance reckless spending of money. Manic episodes lead to marked impairment of social or occupational functioning. In contrast to manic episodes are depressive episodes, which are characterized by vital sadness, anhedonia, low self-esteem, reduced activity, loss of energy, listlessness, as well as reduced concentration. Yet elevated activity in line with agitated depression is possible. Another feature of depression is disturbance of sleep, especially insomnia, early awaking and disruption of sleep. Usually appetite is reduced, whereas also hyperphagia can occur in atypical depression or seasonal affective disorder. Further devastating symptoms are the inability of making decisions, loss of interests and social retraction, even social isolation might occur. Suicide ideation may arise in major depression, as well as suicide attempts and suicide in the last resort [Nabuco de Abreu et al. 2009; Hyong et al. 2008; Kapfhammer et al. 2008]. The change of depressive episodes with marked manic episodes is diagnosed as bipolar I disorder while a change of hypomania and depression is classified as bipolar II disorder in DSM-IV. Hypomanic states are milder and do not cause impairment. Courses of manic disease without depressive episodes are rare [Schulte-Körne 2008; Barnett 2009]. A special subtype of bipolar disorder is called rapid cycling and is defined by switching of mood episodes (depression, mania and hypomania), to remission or to the opposite pole within short time periods. Rapid cycling is characterized by at least 4 episodes within 12 months by DSM-IV. Patients with ultra rapid cycling might even switch within days and ultra ultradian rapid cycler within hours [Bauer et al. 2008; Barnett et al. 2009].

1.1.2 Pharmacotherapy

Psychopharmacological therapy of bipolar disorder is primarily based on mood stabilization with either Lithium or antiepileptics or antipsychotics. Severe acute mania might also need additional sedating benzodiazepines (e.g. Lorazepam, up to 15mg per day necessary in acute mania; usual daily dose 1 10mg per day) temporary. But supplementary use of benzodiazepines should be considered cautiously, because they bear the risk of addiction. In severe depressed states additional antidepressant therapy might be unavoidable. Nevertheless, mild episodes of depression should be treated only by mood stabilizers and non-pharmacological therapy (e.g. behavior therapy, sports and ergotherapy), because antidepressants bear the risk of switching from depressed to manic states and should be considered carefully. Since guidelines change with the current scientific knowledge we want to refer to the following other sources [Benkert and Hippius 2011]:

1. A very detailed version of the treatment guidelines for bipolar disorder by the DGBS („Deutsche Gesellschaft für Bipolare Störungen") and DGPPN („Deutsche Gesellschaft für Psychiatrie, Psychotherapie und Nervenheilkunde") of May 2012:
   http://www.leitlinie-bipolar.de/wp-content/uploads/2012/10/S3_Leitlinie-Bipolar_V1_5.pdf
2. Download of the current "ÖGBP Konsensus Statements" by the ÖGBP („Österreichische Gesellschaft für Neuropsychopharmakologie und Biologische Psychiatrie"):
   http://www.medizin-medien.at/dynasite.cfm?dsmid=58914
3. CANMAT ("Canadian Network for Mood and Anxiety Treatments") guidelines:
   http://www.canmat.org/guides.php
4. Guidelines of the APA ("American Psychiatric Association"):
   http://psychiatryonline.org/guidelines.aspx
5. Last but not least we recommend current editions of psychopharmacological books (e.g. Benkert, Hippius; "Kompendium der Psychiatrischen Pharmakotherapie, 8.Auflage, Springer Verlag") for further detailed information, since we give only a short summary here.

Mood Stabilization

Lithium

Lithium has been the gold standard of mood stabilization since 1949 and is efficient for acute and prophylactic treatment in bipolar disorder, beside it has suicide prophylactic effects [López-Muñoz et al. 2007; Fountoulakis et al. 2010]. One mechanism of action is the influence towards signal transduction systems. One target is the inositolphosphatepathway. Phosholipase C catalyzes the building of inositoltriphosphate and diacylglycerol. Those second messengers lead to activation of proteinkinase C (PKC), as well as intracellular calcium release from the endoplasmatic reticulum. Finally calcium mediates several effects like synthesis and release of monoaminergic neurotransmitters. Lithium inhibits proteinkinase C and influences adenylylcyclase and G-proteins. Furthermore Lithium and antiepileptics inhibit the inositolmonophosphatase, which consequently leads to depletion of inositol. Lithium also shows neuroprotective effects and seems to induce neurogenesis. Beside Lithium inhibits voltage-gated sodium-channels like many antiepileptics (Valproinacid, Carbamazepine and Lamotrigine). Lithium, as well as antiepileptics, enhance the GABAergic neurotransmission and strengthen the serotonergic neurotransmission [Benkert and Hippius 2011]. Lithium is also a potent inhibitor of glycogen-synthase-kinase-3 (GSK3), which is a serine–threonine kinase that intermediates various intracellular signaling pathways [Bhat et al. 2004]. GSK3b phosphorylates and stabilizes the orphan nuclear receptor Rev-erba, a negative component of the circadian clock. Lithium treatment of cells leads to rapid proteasomal degradation of Rev-erba and activation of the clock gene ARNTL. Interestingly Arntl heterodimers with the clock protein Npas2 and the dimer binds to promoter e-boxes of MAOA, which leads to transcription of MAOA. Finally the expressed enzyme mono-amine-oxidase-A inactivates dopamine [Yin et al. 2006]. Since mechanisms of Lithium's antimanic effects are not totally clear, a genome wide association study tried to discover genes involved in Lithium response. They found an involvement of GRIA2, a glutamate/alpha-amino-3-hydroxy-5-methyl-4-isoxazolpropionate (AMPA) receptor gene. Nevertheless, further investigation is necessary [Perlis et al. 2009].

In acute mania the Konsensus Statement of the ÖGPB has recommended a "loading dose" of 900mg Lithium per day. Lithium-concentrations from 1,0 till 1,2mmol/L should be reached in acute mania. The recommended daily dose of Lithium lies between 600 and 1200mg in acute states of mania. Severe acute mania might need addition of antipsychotics or transiently benzodiazepines, because Lithium shows initially given a latency of some weeks. Mild or moderate acute states of mania can be treated with Lithium monotherapy [Benkert and Hippius 2011]. Side effects of Lithium are nausea, tremor, tiredness, polyuria, vertigo, obstipation or diarrhea, weight gain, edema, alopezia, sexual dysfunction, acne, cognitive deficits, arrhythmia or ECG changes in general, hypothyroidism or nephrotoxicity, which can range from mild reduced kidney function till diabetes insipidus, nephrotic syndrome or renal failure [Anditsch et al. 2009; Benkert et al.2011; DGPPN guidelines 2012]. Because of the small therapeutic index, symptoms of beginning intoxication like tremor, vertigo, diarrhea, enhanced reflexes and disorientation over 1,6mmol/L can be expected. Typical symptoms of Lithium intoxication (over 2,5mmol/L) are neurological symptoms, epileptic seizure and dysrhythmia [Konsensus Statement ÖGPB 2008]. Mild Lithium intoxication (1,5-2,0 mmol/L) can be treated by intravenous application of physiologic salt solution and Sodium substitution for increasing the renal Lithium clearance. Severe intoxications (over 2,0 mmol/L) need hemodialysis. Increased effect of Lithium may be due to reduced Lithium clearance and reduced renal perfusion via reduced sodium intake, non-steroidal antiphlogistics (e.g. Diclofenac), Metronidazol, ACE-inhibitors, tetracyclics or diuretics [Rothenhäusler et al. 2004]. Before beginning a Lithium therapy the following analyses are necessary: complete blood count, renal function parameters, thyroid values, blood pressure, ECG, thyroidal investigation, pregnancy test and measuring of weight [Rothenhäusler et al. 2004]. Since patients with bipolar disorder response differently to Lithium treatment, the "ConLiGen-Consortium" was formed to investigate the relationship between SNPs of susceptibility genes and treatment outcome, in a large GWAS with 1200 bipolar patients [Schulze et al. 2010].

Antiepileptics

Antiepileptics (Valproinacid, Carbamazepine and Lamotrigine) inactivate voltage-gated sodium-channels. Beside they influence many signaltransduction pathways similar to Lithium e.g. they inhibit proteinkinase C. Depletion of inositol seems to be a shared effect as well [Benkert and Hippius 2011]. The ÖGPB Konsensus Paper states, that Carbamazepine (e.g. Neurotop®, Tegretol®) and Valproinacid (e.g. Convulex® and Depakine®) are good alternatives for the gold standard Lithium. Both are approved for treatment of acute mania, as well as prophylaxis. If monotherapy is not potent enough the combination Lithium and Valproinacid is recommended. Severe acute mania might need early addition of antipsychotics to antiepileptics. Lamotrigine and Carbamazepine are not admitted for treatment of acute mania, but for prevention of affective episodes. Lamotrigine prevents depressed episodes in bipolar disorder. Interestingly Lamotrigine is supposed to mediate its antidepressant effects among other things via BDNF [Benkert and Hippius 2011; Li et al. 2011]. Side effects of Valproinacid are nausea and vomiting, vertigo, tremor, elevated liver parameter, weight gain, pancreatitis, hair loss, thrombocytopenia, polycystic ovary syndrome and SLE. Valproinacid shows superior onset of action than Lithium and better tolerability with the same efficacy. Therapy with Valproinacid should begin with a loading dose of typically 1000mg per day (exactly 20-30mg/kg body weight). Then the recommended daily dose of Valproinacid for treatment of acute mania lies between 1200 and 3000mg. The maximum daily dose is 3000mg. Therapeutic serum levels of Valproinacid should be between 75 and 120 µg/ml. Side effects of Carbamazepine are sedation, vertigo, ataxia, nausea, tremor, hyponatraemia, allergic reactions, leucopenia, thrombopenia, aplastic anaemia and elevation of liver enzymes, as well as hepatitis. Carbamazepine should be dosed between 600 and 1200mg per day in acute mania. Plasma levels of Carbamazepine from 6 to 12ng/ml should be reached. The maximum daily dose of Carbamazepine is 3000mg. Furthermore Carbamazepine shows interactions with Phenobarbital, Primidone, Zidovudine, Carbamazepine, Lamotrigine, anticoagulans, which increase the plasma levels. The suggested daily dose of Lamotrigine lies between 12,5 and 500mg. The maximum daily dose is 700mg. A slow increase of Lamotrigine is necessary to prevent severe skin reactions (week 1 and 2: 25mg per day, week 3 and 4: 50mg per day, then increase of 50-100mg per 2 weeks). Side effects of Lamotrigine (e.g. Lamictal®) are severe skin reactions (e.g. Stevens-Johnsons-Syndrom), blood count changes, diplopia, tiredness, nausea and vertigo. Furthermore Lamotrigine shows interaction with CYP3A4 inductors (decrease of plasma level), as well as Valproinacid (increase of plasma level, cave: skin reaction) [Anditsch et al. 2009; Konsensus Statement ÖGPB 2008; Fountoulakis et al. 2010; Benkert and Hippius 2011]. Other anticonvulsants (like Gabapentin, Levetiracetam, Oxcarbazepine, Tiagabine, Topiramate and Zonisamide) show more or less positive results in case reports and small studies, but do not have the admission for treatment of mania [Anditsch et al. 2009; Benkert and Hippius 2011].

Atypical Antipsychotics

Atypicical antipsychotics are dopamine receptor inhibitors and have been widely used in therapy of schizophrenia. However, nowadays they are also established in mood stabilization in bipolar disorder. Antimanic effects of Aripiprazole (e.g. Abilify®), Olanzapine (e.g. Zyprexa®), Quetiapine (e.g. Seroquel®), Risperidone (e.g. Risperdal®), Ziprasidone (e.g. Zeldox®) have been shown in several studies against placebo. All atypical antipsychotics are admitted in treatment of acute mania, while Aripiprazole, Olanzapine and Quetiapine are admitted for prevention of manic states too. While only Quetiapine is admitted in prophylaxis of manic, as well as depressed states. In contrast Ziprasidone is the only approved antipsychotic drug for mixed states. Antipsychotics are also especially recommended in dysphoric mania, as well as severe mania with psychotic symptoms. Combination therapies with atypical antipsychotics and Lithium or atypical antipsychotics and Valproinacid are more potent than Lithium- or Valproinacid-monotherapy in severe mania [Benkert and Hippius 2011]. Furthermore the side effects are responsible for choosing the right antipsychotic agent. Side effects of antipsychotics are generally spoken anticholinergic effects (e.g. obstipation or urinary retention), hyperprolactinemia, weight gain, metabolic syndrome, extrapyramidal side effects and very seldom malignant neuroleptic syndrome (the latter shows extrapyramidal effects e.g. akinesia, rigor; hyperthermia; tachycardia; mutism, catatonia, disturbance of consciousness, rhabdomyolysis). Extrapyramidal side effects like akinesia (inability to initiate movement), akathisia (feeling of motor restlessness), acute dystonic reactions (e.g. muscular spasms of tongue; torticollis; oculogyric crisis), pseudoparkinsonism and tardive dyskinesia (involuntary asymmetrical movements of the muscles) have been common in patients treated with first generation antipsychotics (e.g. Haloperidole). But second generation antipsychotics lead rarely to these severe side effects. Nevertheless there are ways to resolve or milden extrapyramidal side effects (e.g. according to the symptom anticholinergic agents like Biperiden/Akineton® or dose reduction or benzodiazepines). Quetiapine shows virtually zero risk of extrapyramidal signs, but similar to Olanzapine, high risk of gaining weight via increase of appetite. Beside Quetiapine and Olanzapine show the highest degree of sedation, while in contrast Aripiprazole or Ziprasidone do not lead to tiredness. In contrast Aripiprazole shows more often of nervousness, agitation and akathisia [Konsensus Statement ÖGPB 2008; Fountoulakis et al. 2010]. The following daily doses are recommended in acute mania: 15-30 mg Aripiprazole, 10-20mg Olanzapine, 400-800mg Quetiapine, 2-6mg Risperidone, 80-160mg Ziprasidone. Interactions: Olanzapine shows interactions with CYP1A2-inhibitors and anticholinergic agents (plasma level increase), as well as CYP1A2-inductors (reduced plasma level). Quetiapine shows interactions with CYP3A4-inductors (decrease of plasma level) and CYP3A4-inhibitors like HIV-protease-inhibitors, antifungal agents, Erythromycin, Clarithromycin and Nefazodone (increase of plasma levels). Aripiprazole shows enhanced plasma levels if given with CYP2D6-inhibitors or CYP3A4-inhibitors, as well as reduced plasma levels if combined with CYP3A4-inductors. Risperidone shows the risk of serotonin-syndrom if given with serotonergic agents. Beside Risperidone shows enhanced risk of akathisia in combination with Fluoxetine, Fluvoxamine and Paroxetine. Like other antipsychotics it shows the risk of hypotonia together with antihypertensives. Antipsychotics also enhance the risk of arrhythmias if given with QTc-time-increasing agents like Amiodarone, Sotalol, Erythromycin, Clarithromycin, antimycotics, Methadone, triptans, 5-HT3-antagonists and others [Anditsch et al. 2009; Benkert and Hippius 2011].

Antidepressant Therapy

Antidepressants helped to release numerous suffering people from the burden of depression. Although antidepressants lead to recoverment for the bigger part of patients, around 30-40% of the individuals do not show full response. It is also difficult to dose antidepressants ideally, because patients with bipolar disorder are at risk to switch from depressive to manic states. Especially potent dual acting antidepressants like NASSA and NARI, as well as older tricyclic or tetracyclic antidepressants show high risk for switching. Instead SSRI and NDRI should be favored. If possible, mild depressive episodes should only be treated by mood stabilizers and psychotherapy. Since patients show various responses to psychopharmacological treatment, genetic profiles might help to create optimal individual treatment plans in future directions [Benkert and Hippius 2011; Konsensus Statement ÖGPB 2008; Kato et al. 2009].

Selective Serotonin Reuptake Inhibitors (SSRI)

SSRI inhibit the serotonin transporter (encoded by the gene SERT on 17q11.1-q12), which mediates the active transport of serotonin into neurons, enterochromaffin cells, platelets and other cells. In the central nerve system the transporters are located in perisynaptic membranes of nerve terminals and dendritic arbors in close proximity to serotonin-containing cell bodies in the midbrain and brain stem raphe nuclei [Murphy et al. 2004]. The serotonin transporter mediates the quick removal of serotonin in the synaptic gap after neuronal stimulation. Blockage of the transporter by SSRI leads to longer maintenance of serotonin in the synaptic gap, because reuptake into presynaptic vesicles is not possible. Potent serotonin reuptake inhibitors (SSRIs) include Fluoxetine (e.g. Fluctine®, Mutan®; daily dose: 20-60mg), Fluvoxamine (e.g. Floxyfral®; daily dose 100-300mg), Paroxetine (e.g. Seroxat®; daily dose: 20-50mg), Sertraline (e.g. Tresleen®, Gladem®; daily dose: 50-200), Citalopram (e.g. Seropram®; daily dose: 20-60mg) and Escitalopram (e.g. Cipralex®; daily dose: 10-20mg). Side effects of SSRI are nervousness, sleeping disorder (especially in the first two weeks), platelet aggregation inhibition, nausea, headaches, loss of appetite, sexual dysfunction, hyponatraemia and QT-prolongation [Rothenhäusler et al. 2004; Anditsch et al. 2009; Kapfhammer et al. 2008; Konsensus Statement ÖGPB 2008; Benkert and Hippius 2011].

NASSA (Noradrenaline and Serotonin Specific Antidepressant)

Mirtazapine (e.g. Remeron® and Mirtabene®; daily dose: 30-45mg), a sedative antidepressant, leads via inhibition of central α_2-receptors and inhibition of negative feedback loops, which usually inhibit the release of the neurotransmitters, to better availability of noradrenaline and serotonine in the synaptic gap. Furthermore it inhibits 5-HT_2 and 5-HT_3 receptors, as well as the H_1 receptor. The latter is responsible for the sedating effect. Common side effects are increased appetite, weight gain, tiredness and headaches. Rare side effects are hypotension, vertigo, nausea, tremor, dry mouth, edema and nightmares. Beside Mirtazapine can lead to increase of liver enzymes, blood count changes and exanthema seldom

[Rothenhäusler et al. 2004; Kapfhammer et al. 2008; Konsensus Statement ÖGPB 2008, Benkert and Hippius 2011].

SNRI (Serotonin and Noradrenaline Reuptake Inhibitor)

Duloxetine (e.g. Cymbalta®, daily dose: 60-120mg), Milnacipran (e.g. Ixel®; daily dose: 100-200mg) and Venlafaxine (e.g. Efectin®; daily dose: 75-375mg) lead to reuptake inhibition of serotonin and noradrenaline and consequently to a potent antidepressant effect with a latency of around 2-3 weeks (antidepressants show a latency of action in general). As mentioned before, the risk of switching is possible. Additionally, common side effects include headache, sweating and nausea. Beside less common side effects are palpitations, sexual dysfunction, loss of appetite, obstipation, nervousness, tremor, insomnia, hypertension, as well as hyponatraemia and QT-prolongation to a minor degree [Rothenhäusler et al. 2004; Anditsch et al. 2009; Kapfhammer et al. 2008; Konsensus Statement ÖGPB 2008].

NARI (Noradrenaline Reuptake Inhibitor)

NARI are a special group of antidepressants, which lead to reuptake inhibition of noradrenaline (e.g. Reboxetine-Edronax®, daily dose: 8-12mg). Side effects are insomnia, agitation and hyponatraemia, as well as pseudo-anticholinergic symptoms. Beside it increases the risk of epileptic seizure [Rothenhäusler et al. 2004; Kapfhammer et al. 2008; Konsensus Statement ÖGPB 2008; Anditsch et al. 2009; Benkert and Hippius 2011].

SRE (Serotonin Reuptake Enhancer)

Tianeptine (e.g. Stablon®; daily dose: 37,5mg) is a serotonin reuptake enhancer, which consequently leads to a balanced serotonin transmission. Side effects are pruritus, headaches, dry mouth, vertigo, hot flash, insomnia- but also tiredness is possible [Rothenhäusler et al. 2004; Kapfhammer et al. 2008; Konsensus Statement ÖGPB 2008; Anditsch et al. 2009; Benkert and Hippius 2011].

NDRI (Noradrenaline and Dopamine Reuptake Inhibitor)

Bupropion (e.g. Wellbutrin®; daily dose: 150-300mg), a noradrenaline and dopamine reuptake inhibitor, leads to less risk of switching compared to SNRI or tricyclic antidepressants. Side effects include loss of appetite, disturbed vision, dry mouth, sleep disorder, headache, tremor, tinnitus, pruritus, sweating, nausea, chest pain, hypertonia and elevated pulse [Rothenhäusler et al. 2004; Kapfhammer et al. 2008; Konsensus Statement ÖGPB 2008; Anditsch et al. 2009].

Tricyclic Antidepressants

Amitriptyline (e.g. Saroten®, daily dose: 100-300mg), Clomipramine (e.g. Anafranil®; daily dose: 100-300mg) and Dibenzepin (e.g. Noveril®; 480-720mg) are not recommended in treatment of depressive episodes in bipolar disorder. They bear high risk of switching, as well as the risk of induction of rapid cycling. Beside those older antidepressants show severe displeasing anticholinergic side effects e.g. dry mouth, obstipation, disturbed vision, tachycardia, cognitive deficits up to delirum (especially in older people); as well as vertigo, edema, hypotension, exanthema, blood count changes and liver enzyme increase. An antidot against intoxication with anticholinergic agents is Physostigmine (Anticholium®) [Konsensus Statement ÖGPB 2008; Anditsch et al. 2009].

Tetracyclic Antidepressants

As well as tricyclic antidepressants, Maprotiline (e.g. Ludiomil®; daily dose: 75-150mg) is not recommended for treatment of depressive episodes in bipolar disorder either [Konsensus Statement ÖGPB 2008]. Another tetracyclic antidepressant is Mianserin (e.g. Tolvon®), which resembles Mirtazapine in mechanism of action. Beside common side effects of antidepressants, Mianserin shows seldom blood count changes (including agranulocytosis), so it is not a first line antidepressant [Konsensus Statement ÖGPB 2008].

MAO Inhibitors

Moclobemide (e.g. Aurorix®; daily dose: 300-600mg), a reversible MAO inhibitor, is not recommended in bipolar disorder as well, as it shows again high risk of switching. Side effects are headaches, dry mouth, sleeping difficulties, nausea, vertigo, agitation, diarrhea, edema and vomiting. Moclobemide shows little risk of hypertensive crisis, since it inhibits predominantly MAO-A (80%). Thus a special diet is not necessary in contrast to the irreversible MAO inhibitors [Benkert and Hippius 2011; Konsensus Statement ÖGPB 2008].

DSA (Dual Serotonergic Antidepressant)

Trazodone (e.g. Trittico Retard®; daily dose: 200-600mg) is a widely used sleep-inducing antidepressant, which is predominantly used to adjust sleeping disorders in affective disorders. It blocks the 5-HT2 receptor, the serotonin transporter, the

$\alpha1$-and $\alpha2$-, as well as H1-receptors. Beside common side effects, the risk of priapism should be mentioned. In contrast it shows no other sexual side effects like libido loss or erectile dysfunction [Konsensus Statement ÖGPB 2008].

Bright Light Therapy

Bright light in the morning leads to a phase advance in rhythms, while admission at night leads to a delay [McClung et al. 2007]. Light administrated in the dark leads to phase delay or advances by activating the circadian oscillator in the suprachiasmatic nucleus in the hypothalamus [Hampp et al. 2008].

1.1.3 Epidemiology of Bipolar Disorder

Bipolar disorder is a serious and devastating disease with a lifetime-risk as high as 1%, some even claim 4%. It is also a destructive disease, because lifetime risk of suicide among bipolar patients is almost 20%. Suicide ideation is common in 14-59% of bipolar patients, and 25-56% committed at least one suicide attempt during lifetime [Abreu et al. 2009]. Mood disorders cause about 1% of all deaths and are one of the society's most important causes of days lost to disability [Michaud et al. 2006]. Manic-depressive disorder is a destroying disease and therefore needs intense research for better insight into biology to invent better strategies against it. In the following chapters genetic insights of bipolar affective disorder will be reviewed. The following part will cover the basic principles of genetics and molecular biology.

1.2 Basic Principles of Genetics

1.2.1 Structure of DNA

Heritable information lies within 46 chromosomes, which consist of DNA that is wrapped around histones. One can imagine DNA as a "spiral staircase" of coding base pair "steps" and a sugar-phosphate backbone. Thus the major three building blocks of DNA are deoxyribose (a five-carbon sugar), phosphoric acid and nitrogenous bases. The treads of the "spiral staircase" are built by flat nitrogenous bases, which pair with each other on the inside of the right handed helix [Langridge et al. 1957; Watson and Crick 1974; Knippers et al. 2001; Lewin et al. 2004]. On one hand there are pyrimidine bases like uracil, thymine and cytosine, and on the other hand derivatives of purine like adenine and guanine. Adenine pairs via two hydrogen bonds with thymine in DNA and with uracil in RNA. The only difference between uracil and thymine is one methyl substituent on position C_5. Cytosine and guanine make three hydrogen bridges. The ability of building hydrogen bonds between base pairs is the reason for hybridization of two complementary DNA strands. The nitrogenous base is linked to position 1 on deoxyribose by a glycoside bond from N_1 of pyrimidines or N_9 of purines. This is how the "steps" are connected to the sugar-phosphate backbone of DNA. The backbone is built by phosphodiester bridges between the deoxyribose molecules, which are the five carbon sugars of the DNA. This means that the 5' position of one pentose ring is connected to the 3' position of the next pentose ring via a phosphate group. This kind of linkage gives DNA a free 5' phosphate end and a free 3'OH end and therefore a direction. Recapitulatory DNA consists of two antiparallel and complementary DNA strands that usually build a right handed double helix with linking base pairs on the inside. Within this simple, but creative construction lies the secret for coding genes and therefore the building plan for proteins, which functions build up the whole complex organism [Watson and Crick 1974; Knippers et al. 2001; Lewin et al. 2004]. Three base pairs (a triplet) code for one amino acid. Thus the key of life lies within the sequence of the bases [Crick et al. 1961]. The sequence of one gene usually codes for one protein or generally spoken for one polypeptide chain. To build the right protein a complex interaction of signal transduction, transcription and protein biosynthesis is needed. Since those mechanisms are very important for the function of our body, those central dogmas of molecular biology will be explained in the following pages [Lewin et al. 2004; Knippers et al. 2001].

1.2.2 Gene Expression- from DNA to Proteins

The first step in gene expression is making a transcript of the template DNA strand, which codes for the protein. Consequently this intermediate mRNA (messenger RNA) is the matrix for converting the nucleotide sequence of DNA into the amino acid sequence of the protein in the second step of gene expression and is called translation or protein biosynthesis [Knippers et al. 2001; Lewin et al. 2004]. Within those complex procedures are many regulation points. Thus gene expression is not a rigid system. Lots of signal transduction signals ultimately lead to protein translation. Genes are the building plan for our organism, but the needs of our body influence how many genes and how often they are expressed. Genes can be transcribed very frequently or they can be silenced via methylation of regulatory elements [Lewin et al. 2004; Bogdanovic et al. 2009]. The following chapter will cover the steps from a gene sequence to the encoded protein. The start of transcription is associated with demethylation and the buildup of an initiation complex. Demethylation at the 5' end of the gene is necessary for transcription, because methylation near the promoter leads to absence of transcription. This is one of the regulatory events at the promoter (the starting point of transcription). An active gene is undermethylated. CpG islands, which can be methylated, are especially located in regulatory targets. They surround some promoters and methylation of those GC repeats prevents transcription initiation [Knippers et al. 2001; Lewin et al. 2004; Yang et al. 2008; Bogdanovic et al. 2009].

Transcription

Transcription is the very first step of protein biosynthesis. As mentioned before, the blueprint of a protein lies in the nucleotide sequence of its gene. Therefore the plan to construct the protein is conserved in the DNA. To express a gene, the enzyme RNA polymerase is synthesizing lots of copies of this DNA sequence. The resulting mRNA represents the coding strand, also called sense strand. Messenger RNA is built by unwinding the DNA-double-helix and complementation of the antisense strand with complementary ribonucleotides (uracil, cytosine, adenine and guanine). The ribonucleotriphosphates get linked by a phosphodiester bond between the ribose (pentose sugar) units under elimination of pyrophosphate. RNA polymerase slides along the DNA matrix in the transcription bubble in 3' → 5' direction of the antisense strand and adds the complementary ribonucleotide to the growing 3'OH end of the mRNA [Knippers et al. 2001; Lewin et al. 2004]. Eukaryotic mRNA must be modified after transcription to be protected during the transport from the nucleus into the cytoplasm. Thus mRNA gets a 5' methylguanosine-cap and a poly(A)-tail. Beside the introns (sequences of eukaryotic mRNA, which are not encoding for a protein) are eliminated during the process of splicing. Recapitulatory the processed and modified mRNA brings the information from the nucleus to the cytoplasm, namely to the protein synthesis apparatus at the ribosomes [Krainer 1988; Tarn et al. 1997; Knippers et al. 2001; Lewin et al. 2004]. The catalyzing enzyme of transcription is called RNA polymerase. Eukaryotes have three types of RNA polymerases [Carter et al. 2009]. Type I catalyzes the transcription of 28S-, 18S- and 5,8S rRNAs, RNA polymerase II transcribes mRNA and Type III synthesizes 5S-rRNAs. Those three enzymes differ in their response to α-amanitin and in their order in chromatography [Knippers et al. 2001; Brueckner et al. 2009]. The structure of eukaryotic RNA polymerases is more complex than those of bacteria. They have at least 12 subunits [Meyer et al. 2009; Carter et al. 2009]. One characteristic feature of the largest subunit of RNA polymerase II is multiple repeats of typical heptapeptides at the carboxy terminal domain (CTD). Those heptapeptides contain serine- and threonine-rests, and are phosphorylated in active enzymes. The phosphorylation is important for the release of the RNA polymerase in the initiation process [Chapman et al. 2004; Knippers et al. 2001; Lewin et al. 2004].

Initiation of Transcription

Transcription can be subdivided into three parts; first initiation, second elongation, and third termination [Brueckner et al. 2009]. Transcription initiation needs a promoter, the starting point for RNA polymerase, as well as helping transcription factors [Chen et al. 2003]. One common element of RNA polymerase II promoters is the TATA-box and it consists of an A-T-rich octamer about 25 bp upstream of the starting point of transcription [Juven-Gershon et al. 2008; Yang et al. 2008; Lewin et al. 2001]. The core sequence of the box is TATAA. Usually it is followed by three more AT pairs and the box is often surrounded by GC-rich sequences. Instead of a TATA box a DPE (Downstream Promoter Element) can be included [Kadonaga et al. 2002; Yang et al. 2008; Lewin et al. 2004]. Another short conserved sequence at the starting point of the RNA polymerase II promoter is the initiator InR [Knippers et al. 2001; Yarden et al. 2009]. In general it can be described as Py_2CAPy_3. There is not extensive homology of sequence at the starting point, but there is a tendency for the first base of mRNA to be an adenine. The InR lies between -3 and +5. In front of constitutively expressed genes ("house keeping genes") are quite often GC-boxes (GpC islands) which can be methylated in silenced genes. Therefore CpG islands are regulatory targets. Methylation of those GC repeats prevents transcription initiation [Yang et al. 2008; Knippers et al. 2001; Lewin et al. 2004]. Beside the typical promoter sequences one can find other gene regulation elements with characteristic DNA motives. Some are around the transcription start and some far away. Regulation elements, which are far away of the start point, are called enhancer [Knippers et al. 2001; Lewin et al. 2004]. DNA-sequence motives are binding places for transcription factors or other regulating proteins. Thus transcription is one possible level of regulation in gene expression. Usually those regulating steps happen around the promoter. Summarized, a promoter of RNA polymerase II consists either of a TATA-box plus InR or an InR plus DPE [Lewin et al. 2004]. RNA polymerase II is not able to bind to its promoter by itself. The enzyme needs a positioning factor to bind to its promoter. The positioning factor is called $TF_{II}D$ and consists of TATA-binding protein (TBP) and multiple TBP-associated factors [Oelgeschläger et al. 1996; Green et al. 2000; Sanders et al. 2002; Knippers et al. 2001; Lewin et al. 2004]. TBP binds to the TATA box in the minor groove. It forms a saddle around the DNA and bends the DNA about 80°. This leads to unwinding of about 1/3 of a turn and to a closer association of polymerase and transcription factors. The outside of the "saddle" is connected to TAFs (TBP-Associated Factors). The largest TBP binding protein is TAF240. This largest TAF is a protein kinase and a histone-acetyltransferase and it is important for recognition of TATA free promoters. TAF240 also represses TBP. Binding of TBP to the TATA box is the first step in the initiation of transcription. Then other transcription factors bind in a defined order. $TF_{II}A$ and $TF_{II}B$ join the positioning factor $TF_{II}D$ (= TBP and TAFs). They stabilize the binding of $TF_{II}D$ to DNA and complete the platform for RNA polymerase II. Actually $TF_{II}B$ builds the surface which is recognized by the RNA polymerase. So this factor is responsible for the directionality of the binding of the enzyme [Kostrewa et al. 2009]. $TF_{II}F$ is a heterotetramer with two types of subunits. One subunit of $TF_{II}F$ binds RNA polymerase II and leads the enzyme to the initiation complex, while the other $TF_{II}F$ subunit has an ATP-dependent DNA-helicase activity. Thus $TF_{II}F$ is involved in melting the DNA at initiation of transcription. However, to really unwind DNA, two other factors are really important namely $TF_{II}E$ and $TF_{II}H$. The factor $TF_{II}E$ leads the very important factor $TF_{II}H$ to the complex. This $TF_{II}H$ factor has several activities. It is a DNA helicase which unwinds DNA at the promoter and it has protein-kinase-activity. With its kinase activity this factor phosphorylates the CTD (the tail of the polymerase with its heptapeptides) which is necessary to release RNA polymerase II from its transcription factor platform and to start the transcription. Altogether this initiation process is quite complicated, but it helps the polymerase to find the promoter sequence, to melt the double strand and to start transcription [Parvin et al. 1994; Nikolov et al. 1997; Wu et al. 2001; Roeder 2003; Lewin et al. 2004; Knippers 2001].

Elongation of Transcription

During elongation the polymerase moves along the DNA, unwinds its helix and extends the nascent RNA chain. Thus new ribonucleotides, which are complementary to the transiently exposed template strand, are linked covalently to the 3'OH end of the growing RNA. This ribonucleinacid is an exact copy of the sense strand and complementary to the template strand. There are only two differences to DNA. RNA contains the sugar ribose instead of deoxyribose and the base uracil instead of thymine. Behind the transcription bubble the two parental strands hybridize again [Knippers et al. 2001; Lewin et al. 2004; Brueckner et al. 2009].

Termination of Transcription

Eukaryotic as well as bacterial RNA polymerases are at least terminated by two possible pathways. Usually RNA polymerase II termination is coupled to transcript cleavage and polyadenlyation for most mRNAs. To a smaller degree also the Nrd1/Nab3/Sen1-dependent pathway can occur. Sen1-dependent termination in eukaryotes is similar to rho dependant termination in bacteria [Peters et al. 2009].

Proteinbiosynthesis (Translation):

Protein biosynthesis is the translation of the genetic code into the amino acid sequence of a protein. This happens in the cytoplasm and needs a protein-synthesis-apparatus which includes tRNA, mRNA, ribosomes, amino acids and enzymes. The mRNA brings the genetic information from the cell nucleus into the cytoplasm to the ribosomes. The ribosomes are the machinery of translation. Eukaryotic ribosomes consist of a 40S subunit and a 60S subunit. The mRNA and tRNA meet at the small ribosomal subunit while the large subunit accommodates the place for knitting the peptide bond [Knippers et al. 2001; Lewin et al. 2004]. The adapter tRNA brings amino acids to the right position on the mRNA via its anticodon. The secondary structure of tRNA looks like a cloverleaf. It has one anticodon-arm, one acceptor-arm, one D-arm and one T-arm. The anticodon of a tRNA is complementary to the codon on the mRNA and consists of three ribonucleotides and represents one amino acid. The acceptor-arm is the "stem" of the shamrock and it is built by the 5' and 3' ends of the RNA, whereas the 3' end overtops the 5' end with three ribonucleotides CCA. The very last ribose of this acceptor-arm-overlap is the binding position of the amino acid which corresponds to the codon in the mRNA. So the tRNA is the adapter for bringing the right amino acid to the right triplet in the mRNA [Knippers et al. 2001]. But the tRNA itself cannot decide, which amino acid belongs to the adapter. For loading the right amino acid on the right vehicle aminoacyl tRNA synthetases are responsible. There is one enzyme for every single amino acid [Knippers et al. 2001; Lewin et al. 2004]. Summarized the tRNA brings the corresponding amino acid via its anticodon to the codon in the mRNA. For every codon there are at least 60 tRNA in one cell, but only 20 amino acids, meaning that some amino acids are coded by more than one triplet. This phenomenon is called redundancy or degeneration of the genetic code. This genetic code is universally valid in every creature of the world [Knippers et al. 2001]. Thus the tRNA anticodon with the very special amino acid docks to the codon of the mRNA in the small subunit. So the tRNA brings the corresponding amino acid to the mRNA and the amino acids are connected by a peptide bond. There are three sites at the ribosome: the A-site, the P-site and the E-site. The aminoacyl-tRNA enters the A-site containing the piece of mRNA with the codon complementary to the anticodon of the tRNA. This makes sure that the right amino acid is at the right place. The peptidyl-tRNA is located at the P-site. The tRNA, which is located at the P-site, has the nascent peptide chain attached. Then the peptide bond is formed between the new amino acid in position A and the growing peptide on the peptidyl-tRNA in the P-site. After the step of knitting the peptide bond the whole peptide chain is attached to the tRNA in site A. One can see the process of making the peptide bond including the transfer of the growing peptide chain to the new amino acid and alternatively to the tRNA with the new amino acid. The formation of the peptide bond is catalyzed by the large subunit. The empty tRNA of the P-site is released via the E-site. After peptide bond formation the ribosome moves one codon on the mRNA. The moving of the ribosomes is named translocation. Alternatively one can imagine the mRNA being pulled trough the ribosome. The process of translocation makes sure that there is always the next codon in the A-site and therefore a new amino acid (the neighbor acid of the amino acid which was knitted to the chain before). So after translocation the tRNA with the grown attached peptide lies in the P-site and the A-site is free again. This makes sure that the order of the amino acids corresponds to the nucleotide sequence of the coding strand of the DNA double helix [Knippers et al. 2001; Lewin et al. 2004].

Initiation of Protein Biosynthesis in Eukaryotes

Protein biosynthesis occurs in three stages: first initiation, second elongation and third termination. Protein biosynthesis starts with the special start codon AUG, which codes for methionine. In bacteria the very first methionine is formylated whereas in eukaryotes only the tRNA of the first methionine differs compared to the carriers of the other methionines within the peptide chain. Beside the start codon, twelve initiation factors are necessary to start translation in eukaryotes. On one hand those factors help the methionine-initiator-tRNA to reach the triplet AUG with its anticodon. While on the other hand the factors help the 40S and 60S ribosomal subunits to meet and connect to the functioning 80S ribosome. About six major steps lead to the complete 80S ribosome and a correctly positioned Met-tRNA$_i$. First of all the small 40S subunit gets prepared for initiation. This happens by binding of eIF1A and eIF3 to the 40S subunit, which blocks a too early attachment of the large subunit to the small one [Kolupaeva et al. 2005]. Then in the second step Met-tRNA$_i$ is placed on the mRNA. The methionine carrying initiaton-Met-tRNA$_i$ and the GTP-binding protein eIF2 build the "ternary complex" which places Met-tRNA$_i$ on the mRNA. This intermediate is called 43S complex, because now the small subunit is heavier and sediments in the ultracentrifuge at 43S. The next step prepares the mRNA for translation initiation. The "cap binding complex" eIF4F binds to the 5' end of the mRNA. It contains eIF4E, which binds to the 7- methylguanosine cap, eIF4A a helicase and eIF4G the "scaffolding subunit". To find the AUG start codon the prepared small subunit binds the 5' end of the mRNA and scans the messenger RNA along the 5' non-coding-region until the small ribosomal subunit finds the start codon. AUG is only identified as the start codon if it is in a special context, the so-called "Kozak-sequence" CCRCCAUGG. The result of this scanning process is the positioning of the small subunit and the initiator Met-tRNA at the start codon. Sometimes this new complex is called 48S complex [Knippers et al. 2001]. The following reaction leads to the exact positioning of Met-tRNA$_i$. The procedure is dependent on the cleavage of GTP in the factor eIF2 within the ternary complex and is organized by eIF5 and eIF5B. Then the used and inactive eIF/GDP and the proteins eIF1A and eIF3 leave the small subunit. Now the blockade of eIF1A and eIF3 of the small subunit is released and the anticodon of the Met-tRNA$_i$ is paired with the start codon AUG. Then the large subunit unites with the small subunit to form the active 80S ribosome. After reunion of the 2 subunits all initiation factors are released and the first methionine lies in the P-site and the A-site is free for the following amino acid [Knippers et al. 2001; Lewin et al. 2004; Pestova et al. 2001; Siridechadilok et al. 2005; Jivotovskaya et al. 2006; Reibarkh et al. 2008].

Elongation

As mentioned before the key process of peptide bond synthesis is based on 3 major steps. First the new amino acid arrives at the A-site with the suiting tRNA-anticodon. In the second step the polypeptide, attached to the tRNA in the P-site (or in the very first step the methionine), is transferred to the new amino acid in place A. The peptide bond is created under elimination of H_2O between the carboxy group and the amino group of two amino acids. And finally, the ribosome moves one codon on the mRNA to generate a free A-site with a new free neighbor-codon and a P-site with the nascent peptide chain. Those steps are repeated until the whole protein-coding piece of the mRNA is translated into the corresponding amino acid sequence. Again, this part of translation needs helping factors. The entry of aminoacyl-tRNAs to the A-site is mediated by the elongation factor eEF1α. Bringing the aa-tRNA to the A-site involves cleavage of the high-energy bond in GTP. The active form is regenerated again by eEF1βγ and changes GDP to GTP. Translocation is coordinated by eIF2. Generally the translocation is catalyzed by the large subunit. Responsible for recognizing the stop codon is eRF [Knippers et al. 2001; Lewin et al. 2004].

Termination

Termination occurs at the stop codons UAA, UAG and UGA. The eRF1 protein is responsible for finding the stop codons in eukaryotes. The eRF1 factor mimics the structure of tRNA. There are no fitting tRNA for the stop codon, thus the peptide chain is completed and released from the ribosomes [Lewin et al. 2004].

1.2.3 Replication

Before cell division, DNA must be copied in the synthesis phase of the cell cycle to give exactly the same genetic material to the daughter cells. Copying DNA happens semiconservatively. This means that the DNA of the daughter cell consists of one DNA-strand of the mother cell and one new synthesized strand. This happens because the mechanism of replication is opening and unwinding the mother-DNA-double-helix and completing each strand with the complementary corresponding deoxynucleotides. The reaction is catalyzed by the DNA-dependent DNA polymerase. This enzyme cannot start by itself therefore it needs a primer with a free 3'OH end. The free 3'OH is very important, because the direction of DNA-synthesis is from 5' to 3'. This means that the DNA polymerase attaches a new nucleotide to the 3' OH end of the growing new strand, which is complementary to the mother strand. This is also the reason why the lagging strand synthesis is performed in short Okazaki fragments. Since the DNA strands are antiparallel, it is only possible on one strand to finish DNA synthesis with only one primer and without a stop. On the lagging strand the replication is discontinuously, because the direction of synthesis is reverse to the fork movement. But since the direction of synthesis is from 5' to 3' and the strands are antiparallel there is always only a short stretch of matrix exposed (from the fork to the next Okazaki fragment). Thus DNA can only be synthesized in short Okazaki fragments, which are connected after excision of the RNA primers and after refilling the gaps with deoxyribonucleotides. On the leading-strand there is always the next necessary matrix of the mother strand (3' to 5') available for complementation, because the direction of synthesis is the direction of the fork movement. So the 3'end of the leading strand can grow along the fork in 5' → 3' direction [Falaschi et al. 2000; Lewin et al. 2004; Kunkel et al. 2008].

Initiation of Replication

Replication starts at the origin. Since the genome of eukaryotes is rather large there are multiple replication origins within the genome. The origin is recognized by the origin recognition complex (ORC). The next step is the addition of Cdc6 and other proteins. In the third step six MCM (Minichromosome Maintenance Proteins) are loaded on the chromatin. They build a ring around the chromatin, which can slide along double stranded DNA. The complex with ORC, MCM2-7, Cdc 6 and Cdt1 is called prereplicative complex (pre-RC) then. The addition of the MCM 2-7 is also called "licensing". A subcomplex of MCM4, 6 and 7 has DNA-helicase activity. This suggests a role in unwinding at the replication fork. The pre-RC adds other factors for instance Cdc45 and Sld3. Now the whole complex is called pre-initiation-complex. The main triggers for initiation are two protein-kinases. One of them is a cyclin-dependent kinase. In metazoans it is CDK2 and acts S-phase-specific together with cyclins A and E [Krude et al. 1997; Lewin et al. 2004; Baltin et al. 2006; Chen et al. 2007; Evrin et al. 2009; Remus et al. 2009].

1.2.4 Epigenetics

Enduring effects of early experience on neural function may be due to epigenetic changes of DNA. Those changes occur without changing the sequence of our genes. Functional changes are created by means of methylation, acetylation and other chemical changes of DNA or histones, which lead to an alteration of transcription and gene expression in general. Thus epigenetic changes influence our body by modifying gene expression. Consequently the blueprint is not changed but the frequency of reading is different. Especially early childhood experiences influence signal cascades, which lead to a change of the "epigenome". This is a possibility how the environment can influence our genome and gene expression, and will be the focus of the following chapter [Oberlander et al. 2008].

1.2.5 Mutations

Gene mutations

Point mutations

Point mutations are gene mutations, which affect only one base pair. Substitution leads to an exchange of one single base in a triplet. Transversion is the substituation of a purine base against a pyrimidine base or the other way round. An exchange of one base against the same kind of base, for example purine base against purine base, is called transition. Since the genetic code is degenerated it is possible, that the changed triplet still codes for the same amino acid. Thus the mutation does not have any effect. However, a point mutation can also lead to a different amino acid. Deletions are more common than substitutions. The deletion of one base pair can lead to a frame shift and to a totally different amino acid constellation. Single Nucleotide polymorphisms (SNPs) are gene variants in a population, which can result from point mutations. One can say those SNPs are "successful point mutations", which established themselves to a certain degree in the gene pool [Buselmaier 2004].

Insertions, Deletions, Duplications and Repeat Polymorphisms

Deletion of some base triplets leads to the loss of the coded amino acids. Yet if the deletion occurs exactly in triplets no frame shift occurs. Otherwise the frame-shift-mutation would lead to totally different amino acids. Duplications lead to a doubled segment or a doubled gene. This can happen during crossing over by mistake. Insertions are the opposite of deletions. Sometimes it happens that one or more base pairs are inserted. Repeat polymorphisms are the amplification of a certain motif, which usually consist of three base pairs [Buselmaier 2004].

Chromosomal mutations

Structural Chromosomal Mutations

Structural chromosomal mutations include deletions, duplications, insertions, inversions and translocations. Terminal deletions result from breaking off the end of chromosomes. While the lost of a part in the middle of a chromosome lead to an interstitial deletion. Large deletions are often lethal, since important genetic information is lost. Translocation describes the changing of position and incorporation of a chromosomal fragment at another place. Inversions are mutations, which result by breaking out of a chromosome segment and reintegration at the same place, but in wrong direction [Buselmaier 2004].

Chromosome Number Aberrations

Whole chromosomes can get lost or added during meiosis. This results in trisomy or monosomy. However, the whole set of chromosomes can be as well either doubled or tripled [Buselmaier 2004].

1.2.6 Methods of Molecular Bipolar Disorder Research

Association Studies

Association studies are important methods to investigate complex traits, for example bipolar disorder. This method detects smaller effect sizes much better than linkage studies. Association studies are usually performed as a case-control design. They search for association between an allele marker and disease within a population, which cannot occur only by chance. The association approach includes comparing the frequency of a gene polymorphism in unrelated affected individuals and a control sample that is representative of the allelic distribution in the general population or totally unaffected individuals, which would be a supernormal group. The case-control design bears the danger of spurious association, because of unsuspected population stratification. This can be avoided in family-based association designs. The non-transmitted alleles of the parents of a singly ascertained patient represent a random sample of alleles from the population and are used as a well-matched control sample. One popular family-based association study method is the transmission disequilibrium test (TDT). It is a test for excess transmission of a marker allele to affected individuals over and above that expected by chance. Family-based association studies have the disadvantage that gene-environment-interactions cannot be examined and that sample sizes are difficult to collect [Craddock et al. 2001]

Genome Wide Association Studies (GWAS)

Genome wide association study (GWAS), also called whole genome association study (WGAS), is an examination of genetic polymorphisms across the whole genome designed to identify genetic associations with complex traits, for instance bipolar disorder. The human genome project made this approach possible. Usually it is performed as a case-control design. The genome of a group with the disease and the genome of a healthy control group is genotyped, in other words, sequenced. Then the detected gene variant frequencies, the occurrence of special markers, are compared between cases and controls with special software. If a certain gene polymorphism is more frequent in the case group, the polymorphism is associated with the disease. GWAS are an excellent way to detect gene polymorphisms associated with disorders without bias of choosing special supposed genes. Furthermore they are powerful to detect even genes with small effect, which is especially necessary in psychiatric genetics. In addition this approach also avoids bias due to population stratififaction. But they are quite expensive on the other hand. Nevertheless this approach is the gold standard of psychiatric genetics nowadays [Pearson et al. 2008].

Linkage studies

Linkage studies seek to identify the loci that cosegregate with a specific genomic region, which is tagged by polymorphic markers, within families. Generally spoken linkage means the tendency of genes that are located close to each other on a chromosome to be inherited together during meiosis, because they are less likely to be separated during crossing over. The relative distance between two genes can be calculated by looking at the way of inheritance and location of two usually linked genetic traits in the offspring and the percentage of disruption of the linkage of two traits. If both traits are not farther away in the offspring in 50% genes can be claimed to be "linked". Genetic linkage can also be understood by looking at the relationships among phenotypes. Among individuals of an experimental population or species, some phenotypes or traits can occur randomly with respect to one another or with some correlation to another. A linkage map is a genetic map that shows the position of its known genes or genetic markers relative to each other in terms of recombination frequency, rather than a specific physical distance along each chromosome. Linkage mapping can be used for identifying the location of genes that cause genetic diseases, but it is an old fashioned approach. In other words a genetic map is a map based on the frequencies of recombination between markers during crossing over of homologous chromosomes. The greater the frequency of recombination between two genetic markers, the farther apart they are supposed to be. The other way round, the lower the frequency of recombination between the markers, the smaller the physical distance between them. Historically, the markers originally used were detectable phenotypes (enzyme production, eye color) derived from coding DNA sequences. Finally confirmed or assumed noncoding DNA sequences e.g. microsatellites or RFLPs (restriction fragment length polymorphisms) have been used. Genetic maps helped researchers to locate other markers, like other genes, by testing for genetic linkage of the already known markers. Newton E. Morton developed the LOD score, a statistical test often used for linkage analysis in human, animal and plant populations. The LOD score compares the likelihood of obtaining the test data if the two loci are indeed linked, to the likelihood of observing the same data purely by chance. Positive LOD scores favor the presence of linkage, whereas negative LOD scores show that linkage is less likely [Griffiths et al. 1993; Morton 1955; Griffiths et al. 1999].

2. Methods

We searched Pubmed with the following key words: History of bipolar disorder; History of schizophrenia; Kraepelin and bipolar disorder; Kraepelin and schizophrenia; Bipolar disorder genetics; genetics and bipolar disorder; pathogenesis bipolar disorder; DNA structure Watson and Crick; Triplet code; DNA is a double helix; eukaryotic transcription; eukaryotic translation; splicing mRNA; types of RNA polymerase; bdnf and bipolar disorder; neurotrophic factor and bipolar disorder; Val66Met allele; Val66Met and bipolar disorder; linkage studies bipolar disorder; BDNF and functions; BDNF and neurogenesis; BDNF and neuron growth; COMT and bipolar disorder; COMT and affective mood disorder; Catechol-O Methyltransferase and bipolar disorder; MAO gene and bipolar disorder; MAO-A gene bipolar disorder; MAO-A gene association studies bipolar affective disorder; clock genes and bipolar disorder; Arntl and bipolar disorder; Arntl and mood disorder; Bmal1 mania; Mop3 mania; Arntl mania; clock bipolar disorder; suprachiasmatic nucleus; circadian oscillator genes; mammalian circadian oscillator; NR1D1 and bipolar disorder; CLOCK gene and bipolar disorder; animal study of clock genes and bipolar disorder; association studies of clock genes and bipolar disorder; Dbp bipolar disorder; Serotonergic genes and bipolar disorder; serotonergic receptor genes and bipolar disorder; (5-HT)-receptor genes; HTR1; HTR2A and bipolar affective disorder; HTR3 and bipolar affective disorder; HTR3 and mania; 5-HT receptor and bipolar disorder; HTR4 and bipolar disorder; HTR5 and bipolar disorder; HTR6 and bipolar disorder; HTR7 and bipolar disorder; serotonin transporter and bipolar disorder; serotonin transporter promoter region and bipolar disorder; 5HTTLPR and bipolar disorder; VNTR and bipolar disorder; SERT and bipolar disorder; CACNA1C and bipolar disorder; CACNA1B and bipolar disorder; ion channel genes and bipolar disorder; KCN2 bipolar disorder; heritability twin studies bipolar disorder. Gene environment interactions bipolar disorder; maltreatment and genotype and depression; BDNF and maltreatment and bipolar disorder; serotonin transporter and maltreatment and bipolar disorder; famines and genes and bipolar disorder; infections and bipolar disorder; serotonin transporter gene and stress; serotonin transporter gene and maltreatment; serotonin transporter gene and stress response; 5-HTTPLR polymorphism and environment; 5-HTTLPR maltreatment bipolar disorder; 5-HTTLPR and life events; CRHR1 linkage bipolar disorder 17q12-q22; CRH and bipolar disorder; HPA and bipolar disorder; 8q13 linkage bipolar disorder; Dopamine system and bipolar disorder; DRD1 and bipolar disorder; DRD2 and bipolar disorder; DRD3 and bipolar disorder; DRD4 and bipolar disorder; DRD5 and bipolar disorder; DAT1 and bipolar disorder; overlaps bipolar disorder and schizophrenia; overlaps bipolar disorder and major affective disorder; overlaps manic depressive disease and major depression; COMT and depression; COMT and schizophrenia; COMT and bipolar disorder; all gene locations were searched with the terms bipolar disorder and linkage studies; all genes in the lists were searched together with the term bipolar disorder; All genes in the lists were searched with the term schizophrenia, major depression and bipolar disorder; All studies until 28thof January 2013 have been included. This book represents the current knowledge of genetics of bipolar disorder.

3. Genetics of Bipolar Disorder

3.1 Heritability of Bipolar Disorder

Bipolar disorder is a highly heritable disease, which has been proven by many twin and adoption studies for decades. Heritability is as high as 80-85% [Cardno et al. 1999; McGuffin 2003]. Concordance rates between monozygotic twins are 40-70% and 5-10% for dizygotic twins. The children of two affected parents have a lifetime-risk of 50-65% to fall ill with bipolar disorder, while children with one parent with bipolar disorder only show a risk of 25% to get bipolar disorder. If one first-degree relative suffers from bipolar disorder, one has the risk of 5-10% to develop bipolar disorder. In contrast people without related affected individuals show a risk of 1% [Rothenhäusler et al. 2004]. This assumes that the genetic constitution is very important for development of manic-depressive disease, but not the only cause. Genetic and environmental factors are the most probable reasons for the pathogenesis of bipolar disorder [Kieseppä et al. 2004].

3.2 Candidate Genes at One View

Since the main model of affective disorders has been dominated by the "neurotransmitter imbalance theory" for decades, it is not surprising that many highly investigated candidate genes have belonged to neurotransmitter systems (serotonergic, noradrenergic, dopaminergic, GABAergic and glutamatergic system) and biogenic amine modulation (e.g. genes encoding for Monoamine-oxidase-A (MAOA), Catechol-O-methyltransferase (COMT) and the Typtophan Hydroxylase 1 (TPH1)). Circadian rhythms are often disturbed in bipolar disorder, so "Clock genes" have been hot spots of research likewise. The growth hormones are another promising chapter of bipolar disorder research as well as genes involved in Lithium signal transduction. The GWAS era elucidated that top susceptibility genes do not primary belong to those classical, expected systems. They are coding for ion-channels (like CACNA1C) or ion channel associated proteins. A detailed description is given in the following chapters [Sklar et al. 2008; Craddock et al. 2009].

Table 1: Candidate Genes for Bipolar Disorder and Supportive Evidence at One View (Candidate genes with at least two significant association study results or two significant linkage study results or one significant GWAS result)

Genes involved in biogenic amine modulation				
Gene	**Location**	**Gene function**	**Significant association**	**No association**
MAOA	Xp11.23	Bioamine degrading enzyme Monoamine-Oxidase-A (degrades noradrenaline and serotonin and dopamine)	Kawada et al. 1995 Lim et al. 1995 Rubinszteinet al.1996 Furlong et al.1999 (meta-analysis) Preisig[1] et al. 2000 Fan et al. 2010 (meta-analsysis in Caucasian)	Nöthen et al. 1995 Craddock et al. 1995 Muramatsu et al.1997 Parsian et al. 1997 Serretti et al. 2002 Lin et al. 2008
COMT	22q11.1-q11.2	Catechol-O-methyltransferase is involved in the inactivation of catecholamine-neuro-transmitters. COMT introduces a methyl group to the catecholamine, which is donated by S-adenosyl methionine.	Lachman et al. 1996 Kirov et al. 1998 Shifman et al. 2004 Funke et al. 2005 Goghari et al. 2008 Abdolmaleky etl. 2009 (epigenetic study) Zhang et al. 2009 (large association study and meta-analysis on 19studies) Lee et al. 2010 Benedetti et al. 2011 Nohesara et al. 2011 (Epigenetic study) Lelli-Chiesa et al. 2011 (BD and emotional progressing)	Gutierrez et al. 1997 Kunugi et al. 1997 Kirov et al. 1999 Geller et al. 2000
TPH1	11p15.3-p14	Tryptophan hydroxylase (TPH) catalyzes the biopterin-dependent monooxygenation of tryptophan to 5-HT which is subsequently	Chen et al. 2008 Bellivier et al. 1998	Lai et al. 2005 Choi et al. 2010 Kwang-Yeon et al. 2010

Genes involved in biogenic amine modulation				
Gene	**Location**	**Gene function**	**Significant association**	**No association**
TPH2	12	decarboxylated to form serotonin. TPH2 is an isoform of TPH that is expressed in the brain.	Harvey et al. 2004 Lai et al. 2005 Van Den Bogaert et al. 2006 Harvey et al. 2007 Lin et al. 2007 Cichon et al. 2008 Roche et al. 2009 Campos et al. 2010 Campos et al. 2011 Grigoroiu-Serbanescu et al. 2010	Mann et al. 2008 Choi et al. 2010 Kwang-Yeon et al. 2010 Serretti et al. 2011
TH	11p15	Tyrosine hydroxylase is responsibe for the first and rate-limiting step in synthesis of catecholamines (it converts tyrosine into L-dopa)	Malfosse et al 1997 Smyth et al. 1997 Craddock et al. 1999 Serretti et al. 2000	De bruyn et al.1994 Muglia et al. 2002 Furlong et al. 1999 Souery et al. 1999

Genes of the serotonergic system				
Gene	**Location**	**Gene function**	**Significant association**	**No association**
HTR1A	5q11.2-q13	G-protein-coupled serotonin receptor distributed in the frontal cortex, septum, amygdala, hippocampus and hypothalamus post-synaptically.	Kishi et al. 2011 Kishi et al. 2012 (meta-analysis)	Curtis et al. 1993 Vincent et al. 1999
HTR2A	13q14–21	Hallucinogens like LSD are agonists to this G-protein coupled excitatory 5-HT2A receptor, while antipsychotics inhibit this receptor subtype. Also involved in contraction of blood vessels and shape changes in platelets; Almost all polymorphisms showed negative study results especially the best studied HTR2A-SNP C102T.	Stine et al. 1997 (linkage study) Badenhop et al. 2001 (linkage study) Ranade et al. 2003 Le Niculescu et al. 2008 (convergent re-analys of GWAS) McAuley et al. 2009 Abdolmaleky et al.2011	Arranz et al. 1997 Gutiérrez et al.1997 Mahieu et a. 1997 Zhang et al. 1997 Tsai et al. 1999 Vincent et al. 1999 Blairy et al. 2000 Heiden et al. 2000 Massat et al. 2000

Genes of the serotonergic system				
Gene	**Location**	**Gene function**	**Significant association**	**No association**
			(Epigenetic study) Ghadirivasfi et al. 2011 (Epigenetic study)	Tut et al. 2000 Murphy et al. 2001 Bonnier et al. 2002 Robertson et al. 2003 Etain et al. 2004 Kishi et al. 2009
HTR2C	Xq24	Activation of the 5-HT2C receptor inhibits dopamine and noradrenaline release in certain areas of the brain. Regulates mood, anxiety, feeding and reproductive behavior	Pekkarinen et al. 1995 Gutiérrez et al. 2001 Lerer et al. 2001 Ekholm et al. 2002 Massat et al. 2007 Wigg et al. 2009	Oruc et al. 1997 Vincent et al. 1999 Meyer et al. 2002
HTR3A	11q23	The 5-HT3 ion channel receptor causes fast, depolarizing responses in neurons and leads to nausea. It is also involved in learning, cognition and emotion.	Niesler 1a et al 2001 Hammer et al. 2012	Niesler et al. 1b 2001
HTR3B	11q23	The 5-HT3 ion channel receptor causes fast, depolarizing responses in neurons and leads to nausea and is also involved in learning, cognition and emotion.	Frank et al. 2004 Yamada et al. 2006 Hammer et al. 2012	Lack of studies
HTR4	5q32	This G protein coupled receptor is located in the alimentary tract, urinary bladder, heart and adrenal gland, as well as the central nervous system. 5-HT4 agonists are also active as 5-HT3 antagonists, such as metoclopramide	Ohtsuki 2002 Lewis et al.2003 Hong et al. 2004 Park et al. 2004 Wellcome Trust Consortium et al. 2007 (GWAS)	Lack of studies
HTR5A	7q36.1	G-protein coupled multi-pass membrane protein, which functions in part through the regulation of intracellular Ca2+ mobilization.	Etain et al. 2006 Cassidy et al. 2007 Birkett et al. 2000 Yosifova et al. 2009	Lack of studies

Genes of the serotonergic system				
Gene	**Location**	**Gene function**	**Significant association**	**No association**
SLC6A4 (5-HTT gene, SERT) VNTR polymorphism in intron 2	17q11.1-q12	5-HTTLPR polymorphism of the serotonin transporter gene (SERT). SERT encodes for the serotonin transporter, which mediates reuptake of synaptically released serotonin. It is inhibited by antidepressants like SSRI.	Collier et al. 1996 Craddock et al 1996 Battersby et al. 1996 Kunugi et al. 1996 Rees et al. 1997 Bellivier et al. 1998 Furlong et al. 1998 (meta-analysis) Kirov et al. 1999 Bellevier et al. 2002	Stöber et al. 1996 Hoehe et al. 1998 Bocchetta et al 1999 Vincent et al. 1999 Olivieira et al. 2000 Saleem et al. 2000 Mellerup et al 2001 Dimitrova et al. 2002 Yen et al. 2003 Alaerts et al. 2009
SLC6A4 (5-HTT gene, SERT) 5-HTTPLPR insertion/ deletion polymorphism (short and long allele)	17q11.1-q12	5-HTTLPR polymorphism in the serotonin transporter gene (SLC6A4= 5-HTT)	Bellivier et al. 1998 Rotondo et al. 2002 Anguelova et al. 2003 (meta-analysis) Hauser et al. 2003 Lasky-Su et al. 2005 (meta-analysis) Meira-Lima et al. 2005 Manchia et al. 2010 Neves et al. 2010 (violent suicide attempts in BD) Sugawara et al. 2011 (Epigenetics analysis in concordant monocygotic twins)	Kunugi et al 1996 Collier et al. 1996 Rees et al. 1997 Esterling et al 1998 Hoehe et al. 1998 Mendes de Oliviera et al. 1998 Geller et al. 1999 Kirov et al. 1999 Serretti et al. 1999 Vincent et al. 1999 Olivieira et al. 2000 Ospina-Duque 2000 Bellivier et al. 2002 Serretti et al. 2002 Mendlewicz et al. 2004 Neves et al. 2008 Vincze et al. 2008 Alaerts et al. 2009 Mick et al. 2009

Genes of the dopaminergic neurotransmitter system				
Gene	**Location**	**Gene function**	**Significant association**	**No association**
DRD1	5q35.1	G-protein coupled dopamine receptor D1, which regulates neuronal growth and development. It also mediates some behavioral responses.	Ni et al. 2002 Severino et al. 2005 Dmitrzak-Weglarz et al. 2006	Del Zompo et al. 2007 Szczepankiewic et al. 2007
DRD2	11q23	G-protein coupled receptor D2 inhibits adenylyl cyclase activity. Concentrated in the basal ganglia, but distributed in the whole CNS with diverse density. Blocked by antipsychotics.	Perez de Castro et al. 1995 Arinami et al. 1996 Li et al. 1999 Serretti et al. 2000 Massat et al. 2002 Zhan et al. 2010 Squassina et al. 2011 Zou et al. 2012 (meta analysis) Hu et al. 2013 (BD and comorbid alcoholism)	Souery et al.1996 Stöber et al.1998 Manki et al. 1996 Sasaki et al.1996 Furlong et al. 1998 Bocchetta et al. 1999 Kirov et al. 1999 Li et al. 1999 Heiden et al.2000 Leszczyńska Rodziewicz et al. 2005 Szczepankiewicz et al. 2007 Lafuente et al. 2008
DRD3	3q13.3	Dopamine receptor D3 especially expressed in the limbic area.	Lee et al. 2011 Lee et al. 2012 (Bipolar II disorder)	Shaikh et al. 1993 Manki et al. 1996 Souery et al. 1996 Piccardi et al. 1997 Kirov et al. 1999 Heiden et al. 2000 Elvidge et al. 2001 (meta-analysis and large case control sample) Leszczyńska-Rodziewicz et al. 2005 Szczepankiewicz et al. 2007 Krelling et al. 2008

Genes of the dopaminergic neurotransmitter system				
Gene	**Location**	**Gene function**	**Significant association**	**No association**
DRD4	11p15.5	Dopamine D4 receptor- G-protein coupled receptor, which inhibits adenylyl cyclase. D4 receptors are blocked by antipsychotics either.	Manki et al. 1996 Serretti 1b et al. 1998 Serretti 1d et al. 1999 Serretti et al. 2001 Muglia et al. 2002 Lopez et al. 2005 Aguirre et al. 2007 Gonçalves et al. 2012 Cosgrove et al. 2012	Perez de Castro et al. 1994 Oruc 1b et al. 1997 Bocchetta et al 1999 Li et al. 1999 Serretti 1c et al. 1999 Serretti et al. 2002 Serretti et al. 2004 Leszczyńska-Rodziewicz et al. 2005
DRD5	4p16.1	Dopamine D5 receptor- G-protein coupled receptor expressed in neurons of the limbic regions.	Asherson et al. 1998 Ewald et al. 1998	Kirov et al. 1999 Muir et al. 2001
DAT1 (SLC6A3)	5p15	Dopamine transporter mediates reuptake of dopamine, as well as noradrenaline to a minor degree. Target of some antidepres-sants.	Keikhaee et al 2005 Ohadi et al. 2007 Cosgrove et al. 2012 Greenwood et al. 2012	Bocchetta et al 1999 Souery et al. 1996 Kirov et al. 1999 Heiden et al. 2000 Georgieva et al. 2002

Channelopathies and ion channel associated proteins				
Gene	**Location**	**Gene function**	**Significant association**	**No association**
ANK3	10q21	Ankyrin G is an adaptor protein, which regulates the assembly of voltage-gated sodium channels at axon initial segments. Furthermore it plays a role in neurogenesis and neuroprotection.	Segurado et al. 2003 (meta-analysis of genome scans) Baum et al. 2008 (GWAS) Ferreira et al. 2008 (GWAS, P = 9.1 x 10(-9)) Scott et al. 2009 (meta-analysis of GWAS) Schulze et al. 2009 Smith et al. 2009 (GWAS) Lee et al. 2011	Lack of studies

Channelopathies and ion channel associated proteins				
Gene	**Location**	**Gene function**	**Significant association**	**No association**
			(GWAS) Takata et al. 2011 Gella et al. 2011 Chen et al. 2011 (meta-analysis of GWAS) Dedman et al. 2012	
CACNA1C	12p13.3	Codes for the alpha 1C subunit of L-type voltage-gated calcium channel	Ferreira et al. 2008 (GWAS, P = 7.0 x 10(8)) Sklar et al.2008 (GWAS) Askland et al. 2009 (GWAS) Sklar et al. 2011 (GWAS, genome wide-significance) PGC GWAS 2011 (GWAS, genome-wide signific-ance) Green et al. 2012 (GWAS) Arts et al. 2013 (cognitive functioning in BD) Radua et al. 2012 (emotional processing and BD)	Lack of studies
KCNC2	12q14.1	KCNC2 encodes the Shaw-related voltage-gated potassium channel.	The Wellcome Trust Case Con-trol Consortium 2007 (GWAS)	Lack of studies
P2RX7/4	12q24.31	P2RX7/4 encodes a purinergic ATP-binding calcium channel receptor, which is involved in 2-arachidonoylglycerol production by microglial cells.	Barden et al. 2006 Soronen et al. 2011	Lack of studies

Channelopathies and ion channel associated proteins				
Gene	**Location**	**Gene function**	**Significant association**	**No association**
SLC39A3	19p13.3	Channel for zink reuptake.	Baum et al. 2008 (meta-analysis of two GWAS) Ollila et al. 2009	Lack of studies

Growth hormones, brain development and neuronal growth				
Gene	**Location**	**Gene function**	**Significant association**	**No association**
EGFR	7p12	Epidermal growth factor receptor, which binds Neuregulin1.	Sklar et al. 2008 (GWAS)	Lack of studies
BDNF	11p13	Bdnf is involved in neuronal migration, serotonergic axon growth, synapse formation, neuronal survival and growth. It is also a key regulator of synaptic plasticity and memory. Beside Bdnf has antidepressant effect by itself.	Sklar et al. 2002 Neves-Pereira et al. 2002 Geller et al. 2004 Lohoff et al. 2005 Sklar et al. 2008 Le-Niculescu et al. 2008 (GWAS analysis) Liu et al. 2008 Vincze et al.2008 Xu et al. 2009 Xu et al. 2010 Sears et al. 2011 Ivanova et al. 2012 Wang et al. 2012	Hong et al.2003 Nakata et al.2003 Skibinska et al. 2004 Kunugi et al. 2004 Oswald et al. 2004 Kanazawa et al.2007 Kim et al. 2008 Mick et al. 2009 Grzywacz et al. 2010 (BD and comorbid alcoholism)
NCAM1	11q23.1	Neural cell adhesion molecule 1 is involved in neuronal growth and pathway formation	Arai et al. 2004 Atz et al. 2007	Lack of studies
DISC1	1q42.1	"Disrupted in schizophrenia 1" was discovered, because it was translocated in some families. The gene DISC1 regulates the neuronal progenitor proliferation via modulation of GSK3beta/beta-catenin signaling. It modulates synapse composition and func-	Rubinsztein et al. 1996 Furlong et al. 1999 Blackwood et al. 2001 Thomson et al. 2005 Müller et al. 2007 Palo et al. 2007	Lack of studies

Growth hormones, brain development and neuronal growth				
Gene	**Location**	**Gene function**	**Significant association**	**No association**
		tion, as well as enhancement of synaptic vesicle transport along microtubules.	Hennah et al. 2009 Le-Niculescu et al.2009 Schosser et al. 2010	
NRG1	8p12	Mediates cell-cell interactions and plays critical roles in the growth and development of multiple organ systems. Also involved in schizophrenia predisposition.	Segurado et al. 2003 Green et al. 2005 Walss-Bass et al. 2006 Georgieva et al. 2008 Perlis et al. 2008 Sklar et al. 2008 Goes et al. 2009 Le-Niculescu et al.2009 Prata et al. 2009 Walker et al. 2010	Moon et al. 2011
IGF1	12q23.2	Insuline like growth factor is similar to insulin in function and structure. IGF1 mediates many growth effects.	Pereira et al. 2011 (GWAS, genome wide significance)	Lack of studies

Clock genes				
Gene	**Location**	**Gene function**	**Significant association**	**No association**
PER3	1p36.23	Per proteins associate with Cry1 and Cry2. Phosphorylated Cry and Per protein complexes enter the nucleus and suppress their own transcription by binding Arntl-Npas2 or Arntl-Clock heterodimers.	Nievergelt et al. 2006 Mansour et al. 2006 Dallaspezia et al. 2011	Kripke et al.2009 Shi et al. 2008
ARNTL (Bmal1)	11p15	Arntl heterodimers with Npas2 and bind to promoter eboxes of MAOA. This leads to transcription of MAOA and finally to inactivation of dopamine and inhibition of the promanic effect of dopamine! Arntl also activates the transcription of other clock genes.	Le-Niculescu et al. 2008 Mansour et al. 2006 Nievergelt et al. 2006	Kripke et al. 2009 Shi et al. 2008

Clock genes				
Gene	**Location**	**Gene function**	**Significant association**	**No association**
CRY1	12q23-q24.1	CRY genes code for chryptochromes, which are mammalian circadian photoreceptors in the retina and pacemaker elements of the SCN.	Ewald et al. 2002 Glaser et al. 2005 Green et al. 2005 Cassidy et al.2007	Nievergelt et al. 2005 Mansour et al. 2006 Shi et al. 2008
CSNK1ε		Casein kinase 1 delta and Casein kinase 1 epsilon phosphorylate core genes of the circadian oscillator (Per1, Per2, Per3 and Cry1, Cry2, Cry3). Phosphorylation of PER genes is a speed determining step in the circadian cycle and modulates cycle length.	Nievergelt et al. 2006 Shi et al. 2008	Lack of studies
CLOCK	4q12	A dimer of Clock and Arntl is the main transcriptional activator of many clock genes (including CRY1 and 2 and PER 1-3 genes). Clock and Arntl activate transcrip-tion of REV-ERBa gene. Clock activates transcription of Dbp, another clock gene product.	Shi et al. 2008 Kripke et al. 2009 Soria et al. 2010	Kishi et al. 2009 (Japanese) Mansour et al. 2006 Nievergelt et al. 2006
NRIDI (REV-ERBa gene)	17q11.2	The gene product inhibits transcription of ARNTL, CLOCK and NPAS2. It is a major regulator of cyclic ARNTL transcription. Lithium leads to degradation of NRIDI.	Kripke et al. 2009 Severino et al. 2009	Shi et al. 2008

Genes of the Lithium signal transduction pathway				
Gene	**Location**	**Gene function**	**Significant association**	**No association**
DGKH	13q14.11	Diacylglycerol kinase-η, a key protein in the lithium-sensitive phosphatidyl inositol pathway.	Ollila et al. 2009 (GWAS) Baum et al. 2007 (GWAS, ge-nome wide significance) Baum et al. 2008 Yosifova et al. 2011 (GWAS, modest association) Takata et al. 2011	Tesli et al. 2009

Genes of the Lithium signal transduction pathway				
Gene	**Location**	**Gene function**	**Significant association**	**No association**
			(meta-analysis) Weber et al. 2011 Zeng et al. 2011	
SORCS2	4p16.1	SORCS2 encodes for the "Sortilin-related VPS10 domain containing receptor 2", which is involved in Lithium pathway	Baum et al. 2008 (GWAS) Ollila et al. 2009 (GWAS) Takata et al. 2011	Lack of studies
DFNB31	9q32-q34	Encodes for Whirlin, which is also involved in Lithium transduction pathways.	Baum et al. 2008 (GWAS)	Lack of studies
PDE10A	6q27	Phosphodiesterase10A-Antagonists of the enzym are currently in clinical testing.	Kerner et al. 2011 (GWAS, genome wide association)	Lack of studies
NXN	17p13.3	Nucleoredoxin inhibits Wnt-β-catenin signaling, which is supposed to play an important role in the mechanism of action of mood stabilizing medications	Baum et al. 2008 (GWAS)	Lack of studies

Genes of the glutamatergic neurotransmitter system				
Gene	**Location**	**Gene function**	**Significant association**	**No association**
GRIN2B	12p12	Subunit 2B of the ionotropic NMDA glutamate receptor, which is a ion channel permeable for Na^+, K^+, and Ca^{2+} and is found at excitatory synapses throughout the brain.	Fallin et al. 2005 Avramopoulos et al. 2007 Szczepankiewicz et al. 2009 Dalvie et al. 2010 Lorenzi et al. 2010	McInnis et al. 2003
GRIA1	5q31.1	Ligand gated ionotropic AMPA glutamate receptor.	Herzberg et al. 2006 Shi et al. 2008 Kerner et al. 2009	Chiesa et al. 2012

Genes of the glutamatergic neurotransmitter system				
Gene	**Location**	**Gene function**	**Significant association**	**No association**
GRM3	7q21.1-q21.2	Metabotropic glutamate receptor 3	Fallin et al. 2005 Dalvie et al. 2010	Marti et al. 2002
GRM7	3p26.1-p25.1	Metabotropic glutamate receptor 7	Wellcome Trust Consortium 2007 (GWAS) Alliey-Rodriguez et al.2011 (Neuroticism Anxiety in BD)	Lack of studies
GRIK4	11q22.3	Kainate-type glutamate receptor	Pickard et al. 2006 Pickard et al. 2008	Lack of studies

Genes of the GABAergic neurotransmitter system				
Gene	**Location**	**Gene function**	**Significant association**	**No association**
GABRB1	4p12	Member of the GABA-A receptor gene family of heteromeric pentameric ligand-gated ion channels. GABA-A receptors are the site of action of barbiturates, benzodiazepines and ethanol. Each gene encodes a subunit of the GABA-A receptor.	Wellcome trust consortium 2007 (GWAS) Green et al. 2010	Lack of studies
GABRA3	Xq28		Baron et al.1994 Wigg et al. 2009 Massat et al. 2002	Papadimitriou et al. 2001
GABRA5	15q11-q13		Papadimitriou et al. 1998 Otani et al. 2005	Lack of studies

Signaltransduction				
Gene	**Location**	**Gene function**	**Significant association**	**No association**
GRK3	22q12.1	G-protein receptor kinase 3, which is a beta-adrenergic receptor kinase.	Barrett et al. 2007 Zhou et al. 2008	Prata et al. 2006
PTGFR	1p31.1	Prostaglandin-F-receptor. Activates luteolysis in the corpus luteum and is involved in smooth muscle contraction in uterus.	Chen et al. 2011 (meta-analysis of GWAS and replication, genome wide significance)	Lack of studies

HPA axis and stress				
Gene	**Location**	**Gene function**	**Significant association**	**No association**
CRH	8q13	Corticotropin releasing hormone.	Marcheco-Teruel et al. 2006 Ceulemans et al. 2011	Stratakis et al. 1997 Alda et al. 2000
Cell adhesion				
Gene	**Location**	**Gene function**	**Significant association**	**No association**
TSPAN8	12q14.1-q21.1	Cell-surface protein, which build complexes with integrins and mediates signal transduction events that play a role in the regulation of cell development, activation, growth and motility.	Sklar et al. 2008 (GWAS, P=6.11 x 10(-7)) Scholz et al. 2010	Lack of studies
JAM3	11q25	Junctional adhesion molecule	Baum et al. 2008 (meta-analysis of GWAS)	Lack of studies
PDLIM5	4q22	Scaffold protein that tethers protein kinases to the Z-disk in striated muscles. Functions in cardiomyocyte expansion and in restraining postsynaptic growth of excitatory synapses.	Kato et al. 2005 Shi et al. 2008 Squassina et al. 2008 Zhao et al. 2009	Lack of studies
NCAN	19p12	NCAN, which codes for an extracellular glycoprotein, is involved in adhesion and migration	Cichon et al. 2011 (GWAS, genome wide significance)	Lack of studies
Mitosis, tumorgenesis and DNA repair/DNA stability				
Gene	**Location**	**Gene function**	**Significant association**	**No association**
GNL3	3p21.1	Guanine nucleotide binding protein-like 3 may interact with p53 and may be involved in tumorigenesis	Scott et al. 2008 (meta-analysis of GWAS)	Lack of studies
PALB2	16p12.2	Involved in stability of key nuclear structures including chromatin and the nuclear matrix. Binding partner and localizer of BRCA2. PALB2 links BRCA1 and BRCA2 in the DNA-damage response.	Ollila et al. 2009 Wellcome Trust Consortium 2007 (GWAS, P=6.3×10-8) Ekholm et al. 2003 (GWAS)	Lack of studies

Mitosis, tumorgenesis and DNA repair/DNA stability				
Gene	**Location**	**Gene function**	**Significant association**	**No association**
NEK4	3p21.1	NIMA related kinase 4, which seems to be involved in microtubule association in mitosis.	Scott et al. 2008 (meta-analysis GWAS)	Lack of studies
BRCA2	16p12.2	Involved in maintenance of genome stability, specifically via the homologous recombination pathway for double-strand DNA repair	Ekholm et al. 2003 (GWAS) Wellcome Trust Consortium 2007 (GWAS) Ollila et al. 2009 Tesli et al. 2010	Lack of studies

Others				
Gene	**Location**	**Gene function**	**Significant association**	**No association**
G72/G30 (DAOA)	13q13-q14	Involved in mitochondrial function and dendritic arborization. Activator of D-amino acid oxidase, which degrades the gliotransmitter D-serine, an activator of NMDA type glutamate receptors.	Fallin et al. 2005 Schulze et al. 2005 Bass et al. 2009 Maziade et al. 2009 Grigoroiu-Serbanescu et al. 2010 Müller et al. 2011	Shi et al. 2008 Gomez et al. 2009 Maheshwari et al. 2009
CHMP1.5	18p11.2	Chromatin modifying protein 1B	Detera-Wadleigh et al. 1999 Segurado et al. 2003 (meta-analysis of genome scans)	McNabb et al. 2005
GCHI	14q22-24	Rate-limiting enzyme in the biosynthesis of tetrahydrobiopterin, a natural cofactor for tyrosine and tryptophan hydroxylase.	Lau et al. 2003 Kaeley et al. 2005 Cassidy et al. 2007 (GWAS) Zhao et al. 2007 (GWAS)	Lack of studies
NAPG	18p11	Soluble NSF, which seem to belong to the intracellular membrane fusion apparatus.	Weller et al. 2006 Li et al. 2009	Li et al. 2012
MYO5B	18q21	Encodes for myosin, which is involved in plasma membrane recycling	Sklar et al. 2008 (GWAS, strongest association within GWAS, P=1.56x10(-7))	Lack of studies

Others				
Gene	**Location**	**Gene function**	**Significant association**	**No association**
SYN3	22q12.3	Member of the synapsin gene family. Neuronal phosphoproteins which associate with the cytoplasmic surface of synaptic vesicles.Role in synaptogenesis.	Lachman et al.2006 (for Czech sample) Wellcome Trust Consortium 2007 (GWAS, P=7.2 × 10-5)	Lack of studies
DTNBP1	6p22.3	Dysbindin has a role in organelle biogenesis and is associated with melanosomes, platelet dense granules and lysosomes	Fallin et al. 2005 Breen et al. 2006 Pae et al. 2007 Joo et al. 2007 Corvin et al. 2008 Gaysina 2009	Raybould et al. 2005
TRANK1 (LBA1)	3p22.2	"Tetratricopeptide repeat and ankyrin repeat containing protein". Exact function still unclear.	Chen et al. 2011 (GWAS-meta-analysis, genome wide significance) Goes et al. 2012 (meta-analysis of GWAS, subtype psychotic BD)	Lack of studies
LMAN2L	2q11.2	"Lectin, mannose-binding 2-like"	Chen et al. 2011 (GWAS-meta-analysis, genome wide significance)	Lack of studies
MARK1	1q41	MAP/microtubule affinity-regulating kinase.	Kerner et al. 2011 (GWAS, genome wide significance in BD with substance abuse)	Lack of studies
SLC22A16	6q21-q22.1	Carnitine transporter	Fan et al. 2009 (GWAS) Fan et al. 2010	Lack of studies
BRD1	22q13.33	"Bromodomain containing 1"	Severinsen et al. 2006 Nyegaard et al. 2009	Lack of studies
DCTN5	16p12.2	Dynactin is involved in intracellular transport. Interacts with the geneproduct of 'Disrupted in schizophrenia 1' (DISCI)	The Wellcome Trust Case Control Consortium 2007 (GWAS, P=6.3×10-8)	Lack of studies

Others				
Gene	**Location**	**Gene function**	**Significant association**	**No association**
NDUFAB1	16p12.2	NADH dehydrogenase, a subunit of complex I of the mitochondrial respiratory chain	The Wellcome Trust Case Control Consortium 2007 (GWAS,)	Lack of studies
ITIH1	3p21.2-p21.1	Codes for heavy chain of a serine protease inhibitor.	Scott et al. 2008 (GWAS and meta-analysis of GWAS, strongest association)	Lack of studies
ITIH3	3p21.2-p21.1	Belongs to the inter-alpha-trypsin inhibitors (ITI), a family of structurally related plasma serine protease inhibitors involved in extracellular matrix stabilization	Scott et al. 2008 (meta-analysis of GWAS)	Lack of studies

3.3 Genes of the Serotonergic System

The serotonin (5-HT) neurotransmitter system has been proposed as a target for genetic research, because the neurotransmitter imbalance theory has been suggested for decades as a pathogenetic mechanism in affective disorders- The serotonin transporter (5-HTT) is inhibited by antidepressants (e.g. SSRI) with great success. In the late 1970s reduced levels of 5-hydroxyindoleacetic acid in cerebral fluid was found in suicide victims [Cronholm et al. 1977]. Depletion of tryptophan, which is necessary for the synthesis of serotonin, has mood lowering effects as well. Furthermore, depressed patients with bipolar disorder show decreased binding of serotonin transporters in SPECT [Chou et al. 2010]. Altogether, genes coding for elements of the serotonergic system have been top candidates for genetic research and have been investigated in many candidate based association studies [Robinson et al. 2009]. Nevertheless, although serotonin receptor or serotonin transporter genes seem plausible to play a major role in bipolar disorder, recent large genome wide association studies (GWAS) did not show significant genome wide association with bipolar disorder, but positive results of smaller association studies are discussed in the following chapters [Baum et al. 2008; Wellcome Trust Consortium 2007; Sklar et al. 2008; Ferreira et al. 2008; Smith et al. 2009; Djurovic et al. 2010; Lee et al. 2011; Pereira et al. 2011; Belmonte et al. 2011; Cichon et al. 2011; Smith et al. 2011; Yosifova et al. 2011; Sklar et al. 2011; Chen et al. 2011; Kerner et al. 2011; Greenwood et al. 2012].

3.3.1 Serotonin Receptor Genes

5-HT1 Receptor Genes

HTR1A

The serotonergic receptor 1A is coded on the long arm of chromosome 5 (exact location on 5q11.2-q13) [Kobilka et al. 1987]. It is a G-coupled receptor, which is distributed in the frontal cortex, septum, amygdala, hippocampus and hypothalamus post-synaptically. The 5-HT1A receptor is also the predominant autoreceptor in the raphe nucleii that slows down the firing rate of the serotonergic neurons and the production of serotonin. Also the presynaptic 5-HT1A receptors reduce serotonergic transmission through the inhibition of tyrosine hydroxylase synthesis [Savitz et al. 2009]. Animal, postmortem, pharmacological, PET and gene expression studies suggested a role of the 5-HT1 receptors in affective disorders [Lopez-Figueroa et al. 2004; Savitz et al. 2009]. HTR1A knockout mice show anxiety like behavior and avoid stressful situations [Parks et al. 1998; Ramboz et al. 1998; Gross et al. 2002]. PET studies showed higher raphe autoreceptor binding and thus decreased serotonergic neurotransmission in affective disorder [Sullivan et al. 2009].

Promoter Polymorphism -1019C/G (rs6295)

The promoter polymorphism -1019C/G (rs6295), leading to a cytosine to guanine exchange at position -1019, blocks transcriptional repression and leads to increased autoreceptor expression. This results in relatively decreased serotonin signaling in postsynaptic forebrain target sites via increased negative feedback. The G-allele of this SNP was supposed to play a major role in affective disorders, but with distinct results. Lemonde and colleagues showed that the G-allele was significantly overrepresented in depressed and suicidal patients [Lemonde et al. 2003; Wu et al. 2008]. The bigger part of the groups could not replicate any association of this SNP with depression or suicidal behavior [Wasserman et al. 2006; Serretti et al. 2007; Hettema et al. 2008; Illi et al. 2009; Videtic et al. 2009].

G659T Polymorphism

Another rare R219L 5-HT1A receptor variant (rs1800044; G659T) was analyzed in a 426 unipolar patients and 643 healthy control subjects comprising sample. Significant association with major depressive disorder has been detected [Haenisch et al. 2009].

Dinucleotide Polymorphism (CAn/GTn repeats)

In the late 90s Vincent and colleagues analyzed HTR1A, HTR1Dalpha, HTR1Dbeta, HTR2A, HTR2C, HTR7, tryptophan hydroxylase (TPH), and the serotonin transporter (SERT) in 103 patients with bipolar disorder and healthy controls, but could not find replicated significant association with bipolar disorder. However, it showed trends toward association of HTR2A variants and SERT polymorphisms. The dinucleotide polymorphism of HTR1A consisting of ten CAn/GTn repeats was not associated with bipolar disorder either [Vincent et al. 1999].

Relevance for Therapy

Animal and clinical studies suggested desensitization of 5-HT-1A receptors in the antidepressant therapeutic mechanism of selective serotonin reuptake inhibitors (SSRIs). Thus gene polymorphism might be useful for treatment response and medication decisions, because certain HTR1A polymorphisms show better response to antidepressant therapy [Yu et al. 2006; Kato et al. 2009].

HTR1B and HTR1D

Huang and colleagues investigated the G861C polymorphism of HTR1B (6q13) in 394 psychiatric patients (alcoholism, bipolar disorder, schizophrenia and major depressive disorder) and 96 healthy volunteers. G861C was associated with major depressive disorder, but not with bipolar disorder [Huang et al. 2003]. 290 probands with DSM-IV bipolar disorder I, bipolar disorder II and schizoaffective disorder (Bipolar type), as well as their living parents were recruited to investigate the G861C and T371G polymorphisms in a family based approach. Nevertheless, variants of HTR1D are unlikely to be involved in pathogenesis of bipolar disorder [Mundo et al. 2001].

5-HT2 Receptor Genes

HTR2A

HTR2A, which encodes the serotonin 2A receptor, is located on chromosomal region 13q14–21. The widely distributed serotonin 2A receptor is a subtype of the G-protein coupled 5-HT2-receptors. This receptor is the target for LSD and other hallucinogens (agonists to 5-HT_{2A} receptors) as well as atypical antipsychotics (antagonists to 5-HT_{2A} receptors). Chronical SSRI or antipsychotic use lead to downregulation of post-synaptic 5-HT_{2A} receptors and mediate long-term effects [Eison et al. 1996]. Polymorphisms of HTR2A have been associated with schizophrenia and major depressive disorders as well as response to SSRI [Kawashima et al. 2010]. A polymorphism was significantly associated with bipolar disorder in a convergent data analysis of genome wide approaches, as well as in two recent smaller association studies [Ranade et al. 2003; Le-Niculescu et al. 2008; McAuley et al. 2009]. Those positive findings contradict almost all other negative study results [Arranz et al. 1997; Gutiérrez et al. 1997; Mahieu et al. 1997; Zhang et al. 1997; Tsai et al. 1999; Vincent et al. 1999; Blairy et al. 2000; Heiden et al. 2000; Massat et al. 2000; Tut et al. 2000; Murphy et al. 2001; Etain et al. 2004; Bonnier et al. 2002; Robertson et al. 2003; Etain et al. 2004; Kishi et al. 2009].

T102C

The well-studied silent T102C SNP of the HTR2A gene, also referred as *Msp1* polymorphism, results in a thymidine to cytosine substitution at position 102 in exon 1, which does not result in an amino acid change. Results within schizophrenia patients showed positive findings in relationship with this polymorphism [Peñas-Lledó et al. 2007]. Some early studies at the end of the 20th century did not provide evidence for an association with bipolar affective disorder [Arranz et al.

1997; Gutiérrez et al. 1997; Mahieu et al. 1997; Zhang et al. 1997; Tsai et al. 1999; Blairy et al. 2000; Heiden et al. 2000; Massat et al.2000; Tut et al. 2000; Murphy et al. 2001]. Also a Japanese association study comprising 325 patients with major depressive disorder, 155 patients with bipolar disorder and 802 healthy controls could not provide any evidence of association with the four HTR2A markers (T102C, -A1438G, Rs7997012 and Rs1928040) and bipolar affective disorder [Kishi et al. 2009]. The T102C and –1438A/G polymorphisms were also investigated for their relation with bipolar affective puerperal psychosis, but they were not associated with bipolar disorder either [Robertson et al. 2003]. Additionally, suicidal behavior was examined in relation with this polymorphism, but without positive results [DeLuca et al. 2007]. Even genomic imprinting and parent of origin effect at this locus were excluded [Murphy et al. 2001; DeLuca et al. 2006]. Since there was no positive study result at all this polymorphism is very unlikely to be associated with bipolar disorder.

516-C/T

This silent single nucleotide polymorphism in exon 2 of the HTR2A gene was not associated with bipolar disorder in early studies [Arranz et al. 1997; Gutiérrez et al. 1997]. Only one small study comprising 93 bipolar cases and 92 controls by Renade and colleagues suggested association with bipolar affective disorder. Since this polymorphism is not as well investigated as T102C further studies might be useful. Nevertheless, it did not belong to genome wide associated results of recent GWAS either, so the effect on bipolar disorder pathogenesis might be of minor impact [Ranade et al. 2003].

1354C/T

Ranade and his colleagues proved significant linkage and association of bipolar disorder with 1354C/T single nucleotide polymorphism, as well as haplotypes bearing the SNP. Since almost all study results of other HTR2A polymorphisms are negative, this positive association is worth further investigation [Ranade et al. 2003]. In addition this polymorphism was associated with remission and response following paroxetine therapy [Wilkie et al. 2009].

His452Tyr

His452Tyr is a structural polymorphism in exon 3 of the 5-HT_2 receptor and is not associated with manic depressive disease [Arranz et al. 1997; Gutiérrez et al. 1997; Etain et al. 2004].

Thr25Asn

Also Thr25Asn, a structural polymorphism in exon1 of the serotonin receptor, is unlikely to be associated with bipolar disorder [Arranz et al. 1997; Gutiérrez et al. 1997].

-A1438G Genetic Polymorphism

Etain et al. as well as Kishi and colleagues could not find any association with the -A1438G single nucleotide polymorphism and bipolar disorder [Etain et al. 2004; Kishi et al. 2009]. Bonnier et al. analyzed 5-HT2A polymorphism in patients with major affective disorder and detected lower suicidality in carriers of this polymorphism [Bonnier et al. 2002]. Furthermore, this polymorphism was investigated in schizophrenic patients with positive results [Peñas-Lledó et al. 2007].

Table 2: HTR2A Gene Variants and Their Association with Bipolar Disorder (BD)

HTR2A polymorphisms	Association with BD	No association with BD
Polymorphic DNA variation T102C in exon 1 of HTR2A		– Arranz et al. 1997 – Gutiérrez et al. 1997 – Mahieu et al. 1997 – Zhang et al. 1997 – Tsai et al. 1999 – Vincent et al. 1999 – Blairy et al. 2000 – Heiden et al. 2000 – Massat et al. 2000 – Tut et al. 2000 – Murphy et al. 2001 – Robertson[1] et al. 2003 – Kishi et al. 2009
1354C/T	– Ranade et al. 2003	
-A1438G		– Kishi et al. 2009 – Etain et al. 2004 – Bonnier[2]et al. 2002 – Robertson[1] et al. 2003
His452Tyr		– Arranz et al. 1997 – Etain et al. 2004 – Gutiérrez et al. 1997
Thr25Asn		– Arranz et al. 1997 – Gutiérrez et al. 1997
-C516T	– Ranade et al. 2003	– Arranz et al. 1997 – Gutiérrez et al. 1997

HTR2A polymorphisms	Association with BD	No association with BD
Rs7997012		– Kishi et al. 2009
Rs1928040		– Kishi et al. 2009
Rs2224721	– McAuley et al. 2009	

1 this study investigated bipolar affective puerperal psychosis
2 study associated lower risk of suicide in bipolar disorder to this allele

Linkage studies

Although association studies of the HTR2A gene mapped the chromosomal region 13q14–21 were disappointing linkage studies, they prove evidence for linkage of 13q14 to bipolar disorder [Stine et al. 1997; Badenhop et al. 2001]. Also closeby regions like 13q32 were linked to manic-depressive disease in genome wide linkage studies [Detera-Wadleigh et al. 1999]. The region 13q14–21 was also identified in a very recent functional convergent analysis of genome wide approaches by Le-Niculescu in 2008. While there are isolated positive results, the bigger part of the linkage-, association- and genome wide association studies are pretty disappointing up to now. Nevertheless, time will tell whether this locus comprises any connection with bipolar affective disorder at all [Le-Niculescu et al. 2008].

HTR2C Gene

The serotonergic receptor 2C (formerly serotonergic receptor 1C) is coded on chromosome Xq24 and belongs to the family of seven transmembrane domain containing G-protein coupled receptors. It mediates effects including appetite, locomotor regulation, sexual behavior and anxiety via signal transduction by phospholipase C [Roth 1999]. HTR2C knockout mice show hyperphagia and increased locomotor activity, as well as increased susceptibility to epileptic seizures [Tecott et al. 1995; Nonogaki et al. 2003]. Linkage studies suggested involvement of the chromosomal region Xq24 in pathogenesis of bipolar disorder [Pekkarinen et al. 1995; Ekholm et al. 2002]. Also a whole genome scan showed linkage to a large region spanning from Xq24 to Xq28 in a pedigree of childhood onset bipolar disorder recently [Wigg et al. 2009]. Lerer and colleagues showed that Ser23-allele-carriers of the HT2CR cys23ser polymorphism are at greater risk to develop bipolar disorder [Lerer et al. 2001], whereas Gutiérrez' group could only find slight overrepresentation of the ser23 allele in a subgroup of bipolar women, but not in men [Gutiérrez et al. 2001]. Other groups could not show any association with this HTR2C polymorphism and bipolar disorder at all [Oruc˘ et al. 1997; Vincent et al. 1999]. Further, other gene variations were investigated by Meyer and colleagues, including two polymorphic dinucleotide repeats, which are separated by a short spacer in the promoter region of the HTR2C gene. Nevertheless, no association between the microsatellites in the promoter region and bipolar disorder was found [Meyer et al. 2002]. The 5-HT_{2C} gene was also discussed in other psychiatric diseases including suicidal behavior, depression and eating disorders. The HTR2C gene was investigated in suicidal patients, however, with conflicting results. Serretti and colleagues contradict any involvement of this locus in suicide, while Videtic recently found a significant association of a functional polymorphism 68G>C (Cys23Ser) in female suicide victims [Serretti et al. 2007; Videtic et al. 2009]. Serretti also investigated the connection of this locus with psychotic features, again with negative results [Serretti et al. 2000]. HTR2C polymorphisms also influence eating habits and are involved in eating disorders [Pooley et al. 2004].

5-HT3 Receptor Genes

The HTR3 genes (HTR3A, HTR3B, HTR3C, HTR3D and HTR3E) code for the five subunits of the 5-HT_3 receptor, a ligand gated ion channel for Na^+, K^+ and Ca^{2+}. HTR3A and HTR3B are coded on 11q23 and HTR3C, HTR3D, HTR3E on 3q27 [Bloom et al. 1998; Davies et al. 1999; Niesler et al. 2003]. 5-HT_3 receptors regulate many physiological effects, for instance drug induced emesis and nociception and it may play a role in behavior of anxiety and cognitive disorders [Bloom et al. 1998]. Especially HTR3A and HTR3B may have a role in bipolar affective disorder [Niesler et al. 2008]. A missense mutation at the 5' upstream region of the HTR3A gene (C178T) was associated significantly with bipolar disorder by Niesler and colleagues [Niesler 1a et al. 2001]. Further, five rare HTR3A variants were not associated with manic-depressive disease [Niesler 1b et al. 2001]. The rare gene variants of the HTR3B locus (IVS6 + 31C > T, IVS6 + 40C > A and 1386T >C) were solely detected in patients with bipolar disorder, whereas a 3 bp deletion was underrepresented in manic-depressive patients. Thus this deletion might be protective [Frank et al. 2004]. Certain HTR3B haplotypes are important in female depressive disorder [Yamada et al. 2006]. Recently HTR3A and HTR3B polymorphisms (rs1062613, rs1176744 and rs3831455) were investigated in a European Multi-Center-Study of 1804 bipolar cases and 2407 healthy controls and a following meta-analysis of three GWAS (Samples of BOMA-BPAD, WTCCC-BPAD and GAIN-BPAD with around 3500 bipolar patients and 5200 controls in total). A significant overrepresentation of the p.Y129S (rs1176744) polymorphism of HTR3B has been detected in patients with bipolar disorder. Thus HTR3B seems to play a major role in bipolar disorder [Hammer et al. 2012].

5-HT4 Receptor Genes

The 5-HT4 receptor is coded in the chromosomal region 5q32, which showed nominal association with bipolar disorder in genome wide approaches [Lewis et al. 2003; Hong et al. 2004; Park et al. 2004; Wellcome Trust Consortium 2007]. This widely spread receptor is connected to adenylyl cyclase and contributes to dopamine secretion [Bonhomme et al. 1995]. Four rare polymorphisms and a special haplotype of this receptor gene are significantly associated with bipolar disorder [Ohtsuki et al. 2002]. Some haplotypes have also been associated with schizophrenia [Suzuki et al. 2003].

5-HT5 Receptor Genes

The Serotonin 5-HT_{5A} receptor is coded on 7q36.1 and is distributed in the central nervous system. It regulates many physiological and pathological reactions including anxiety, sleep regulation, aggression, feeding and depression [Rees et al. 1994]. Genome wide linkage studies suggested this chromosomal region 7q36 as susceptibility locus for bipolar affective disorder [Etain et al. 2006; Cassidy et al. 2007]. Recently also a Japanese association study showed that the HTR5 gene might be a promising candidate. They showed a significant association of the HTR5A SNP rs1800883 with bipolar disorder [Yosifova et al. 2009]. The 19G/C SNP was proven to be significantly associated with bipolar disorder too [Birkett et al. 2000]. A recent association study showed no association between a SNP of HTR5A (rs1805054) and major depressive disorder [Illi et al. 2009].

5-HT6 Receptor Genes

The HTR6 gene is located on 1p35–36 and codes for the 5-HT_6 receptor, which belongs to the family of G protein-coupled receptors that positively regulate adenylate cyclase. The receptor is mainly expressed in the brain areas involved in cognitive processes [Kohen et al. 1996]. Especially one SNP, which leads to a cytosine to thymine exchange at position 267, was studied in relationship with many neuropsychiatric diseases, but with inconsistent results. An early association study shows that the C267T variant is not associated with mood disorders [Hong et al. 1999]. In contrast Vogt and colleagues found an overrepresentation of the 267C allele among bipolar patients [Vogt et al. 2000]. The CT genotype of the C267T SNP has better treatment response in depressed patients [Lee et al. 2005]. The C267T SNP was discussed to play a role in schizophrenia, again with unequal results, either positive [Tsai et al. 1999] or negative [Shinkai et al. 1999; Vogt et al. 2000; Dubertret et al. 2004]. The C267T SNP was associated with

Alzheimer's disease in a Japanese association study [Kan et al. 2004]. Alzheimer patients showed a 40% decline of neurons expressing the 5-HT$_6$ receptor. This shows an enormous involvement of this receptor in cognitive processes and therefore may play a role in neuropsychiatric disease and may be a new target for cognitive enhancement drugs [Lorke et al. 2006].

5-HT7 Receptor Genes

HTR7 encoded on 10q21-q24 was investigated in a study by Vincent and colleagues, but showed no association with bipolar affective disorder [Vincent et al. 1999].

3.3.2 Serotonin Transporter Gene (= SLC6A4, SERT, 5HTT)

The Serotonin transporter (5-HTT, SERT) belongs to the superfamily of the large-solute carriers (SLC) and is encoded by SLC6A4 on 17q11.1-q12 [Ramamoorthy et al. 1993; Esterling et al. 1998]. The chromosomal region around 17q11.2 reached interest in many linkage studies and genome wide approaches for bipolar disorder [Edenberg et al. 1997; Murphy et al. 2000; Liu et al. 2003; Klei et al. 2005; Ewald et al. 2005; Etain et al. 2006; Thomás et al. 2006]. The 5-HT transporter mediates the active transport of serotonin into neurons, enterochromaffin cells, platelets and other cells. In the central nerve system the transporters are located in perisynaptic membranes of nerve terminals and in dendritic arbors in close proximity to serotonin containing cell bodies in the midbrain and brain stem raphe nuclei [Murphy et al. 2004]. The serotonin transporter mediates the quick removal of serotonin in the synaptic gap after neuronal stimulation and is therefore the primary target of serotonin reuptake inhibitors (SSRI), which block the transporter and lead to longer maintenance of serotonin in the synaptic gap [Murphy et al. 2004]. Its transcriptional activity is regulated by the 5HTT gene-linked polymorphic region (5HTTLPR), a repetitive element in the 5'flanking region located about 1.4kb upstream of the transcription start point. Especially this region has been a hot spot of molecular psychiatric research [Heils et al. 1995; Murphy et al. 2004].

Polymorphism of the 5-HTTLPR and the Untranslated Region

The Variable-Number-Tandem-Repeat (VNTR) within Intron 2

The variable-number-tandem-repeat (VNTR) within intron 2 comprises 9, 10 or 12 copies of a 16 or 17 base pair repeat. The 5-HTTVNTR acts as a transcriptional regulator, whereas the 12-repeat-allele has a stronger transcription inducing ability [MacKenzie et al. 1999]. Some positive findings suggested a relation between this variant and bipolar affective disorder, especially with the 12-repeat-allele [Battersby et al. 1996; Collier et al. 1996; Craddock et al. 1996; Kunugi et al. 1996; Rees et al. 1997; Furlong et al. 1998; Bellivier et al. 1998; Kirov et al. 1999; Bellivier et al. 2002]. Furlong and colleagues pooled 1400 individuals for a meta-analysis after they failed to show association between their small sample and this 5-HTTVNTR, and proved significant association between the VNTR in intron 2 and mood disorder (bipolar and unipolar depression) in their meta analysis [Furlong et al. 1998]. Already 14 years ago the Lancet claimed an existing association between the 9-repeat-allele and unipolar affective disorder [Ogilvie et al. 1996], although this positive result for major depression was not repli cated later [Kunugi et al. 1996; Stöber et al. 1996; Hoehe et al. 1998]. Some studies showed association with bipolar disorder, but could not survive correction for multiple testing, as a study from Vienna [Heiden et al. 2000]. This VNTR was also investigated for its relationship with age at onset of bipolar disorder. Patients with two short alleles tended to get the disease at younger age, whereas patients with at least one 12-repeat-allele were affected later [Bellivier et al. 2002]. Nevertheless, many groups failed to replicate those positive results. Even a new Swedish study with almost 600 participants, which included association analysis, mutation analysis and CNV analysis, showed that the serotonin transporter gene might not be associated with bipolar disorder in the Northern Swedish population at all. Conflicting results might be due to different sample stratification, little power to detect association with SNPs of small effect and different ethnicities [Stöber et al. 1996; Hoehe et al. 1998; Bocchetta et al. 1999; Liu et al. 1999; Vincent et al. 1999; Olivieira et al. 2000; Saleem et al. 2000; Mellerup et al. 2001; Dimitrova et al. 2002; Yen et al. 2003; Alaerts et al. 2009].

Table 3: Serotonin Transporter Gene Polymorphisms and their Relation with Bipolar Disorder (BD)

	Association with BD	**No association with BD**
5-HTTVNTR in intron 2	Collier et al. 1996 Craddock et al. 1996 Battersby et al. 1996 Kunugi et al. 1996 Rees et al. 1997 Bellivier et al. 1998 Furlong et al. 1998 (meta-analysis) Kirov et al. 1999 Bellevier et al. 2002	Stöber et al. 1996 Hoehe et al. 1998 Liu et al. 1999 Bocchetta et al. 1999 Vincent et al. 1999 Olivieira et al. 2000 Saleem et al. 2000 Mellerup et al. 2001 Dimitrova et al. 2002 Yen et al. 2003 Alaerts et al. 2009
44bp Insertion/deletion in the promoter region of SERT	Bellivier et al. 1998 Rotondo et al. 2002 Anguelova et al. 2003 (meta-analysis) Rousseva et al. 2003 Hauser et al. 2003 Lasky-Su et al. 2005 (meta-analysis) Meira-Lima et al. 2005	Kunugi et al. 1996 Collier et al. 1996 Rees et al. 1997 Esterling et al. 1998 Hoehe et al. 1998 Mendes de Oliviera et al. 1998 Geller et al. 1999 Kirov et al. 1999 Serretti et al. 1999 Vincent et al. 1999 Olivieira et al. 2000 Ospina-Duque et al. 2000 Bellivier et al. 2002 Serretti et al. 2002 Mendlewicz et al.2004 Neves et al. 2008 Vincze et al. 2008 Alaerts et al. 2009 Mick et al. 2009

Insertion/deletion in the Promoter Region of the Serotonin Transporter

The second extensively investigated VNTR (Variable Number of Tandem Repeats) polymorphism comprises of 16 repeat elements. Within those VNTR lies a 44 bp insertion or deletion in the area of repeat element 6-8, which results in a short allele or a long allele. This polymorphism lies exactly at the 5'-flanking regulatory region of the serotonin transporter gene, called 5-HTTLPR. The 5HTT gene linked polymorphic region (5-HTTLPR), is a repetitive element of varying length in the 5' flanking region located around 1,4kb upstream of the transcription start point.

The short (s) allele of this polymorphism is associated with low transcriptional activity, while the long (l) allele leads to high transcription and thus high expression rate of the serotonin transporter [Heils et al. 1995; Hoefgen et al. 2005]. So this polymorphism leads to changed serotonin reuptake from the synaptic cleft. The short allele has been significantly associated with major depressive disorder and poorer response to SSRI [Serretti et al. 2004; Hoefgen et al. 2005]. Of course this variant was also investigated for its involvement in bipolar disorder, nonetheless, with diverging results. Many studies, including recent large GWAS, did not find any association between the promoter deletion/insertion polymorphism and bipolar affective disorder [Kunugi et al. 1996; Collier et al. 1996; Rees et al. 1997; Esterling et al. 1998; Hoehe et al. 1998; Mendes de Oliviera et al. 1998; Geller et al. 1999; Kirov et al. 1999; Serretti et al. 1999; Vincent et al. 1999; Olivieira et al. 2000; Ospina-Duque et al. 2000; Bellivier et al. 2002; Serretti et al. 2002; Mednlewicz et al. 2004; Neves et al. 2008; Vincze et al. 2008; Alaerts et al. 2009]. Others showed overwhelming positive results. Especially the short low activity allele (s allele) should influence bipolar affective disorder significantly [Bellivier et al. 1998; Hauser et al. 2003; Lasky-Su et al. 2005; Meira-Lima et al. 2005]. Different results may occur because of lack of statistical power of some studies with small size of participants. However, larger studies show inconsistent results as well. A European multicenter study (539 unipolar and 572 bipolar patients and 821 controls) did not identify any association between affective disorder and the 5-HTTLPR polymorphism [Mendlewicz et al. 2004]. Serretti and colleagues performed a large study to solve the relationship between the 5-HTTLPR polymorphism and major psychosis. They investigated 1820 inpatients (789 bipolar, 667 unipolar, 66 delusional, 261 schizophrenic and 37 not other specified psychotic patients) and conducted 457 controls, but they did not find any association between 5-HTTLPR variants and the disease. Not even a difference in variant frequency between the disorders [Serretti et al. 2002]. Nevertheless, a large meta-analysis of altogether 15 studies (2774 bipolar cases and 3652 controls) showed significant association between the short allele of the 44bp deletion/insertion polymorphism and bipolar affective disorder [Lasky-Su et al. 2005]. Also a systematic review with meta-analysis, which comprised 1382 bipolar participants and 2085 controls, showed evidence of association with this polymorphism [Anguelova et al. 2003]. Conflicting results might be due to the heterogeneity of bipolar disorder, thus some groups concentrated on subtypes of bipolar disorder. A large study on 435 patients with mood disorders including major depression, bipolar disorder and rapid cycling, as well as 456 controls by Cusin and colleagues concentrated on recurrent and rapid cycling mood disorders and found an excess of 5-HTTLPR long alleles in patients with rapid cycling [Cusin et al. 2001]. Also Rousseva and colleagues found an association between rapid cycling, yet with the short s-allele [Rousseva et al. 2003]. The insertion/deletion variant of the serotonin transporter promoter was also investigated for association with age at onset of bipolar disorder, however, with negative results [Geller et al. 1999; Bellivier et al. 2002]. Mick and colleagues also investigated the deletion polymorphism in bipolar I disorder in children of 173 offspring triades; again the results were negative [Mick et al. 2009]. In contrast, an excess of the s-allele was seen in younger bipolar patients with psychotic symptoms [Ospina-Duque et al. 2000]. Another possibility is the association of the short allele with suicidality, which is also a common symptom in bipolar disorder. A study by Neves and colleagues investigated 351 subjects with 77 patients with previous suicide attempts with the conclusion, that the s-allele was not associated with bipolar disorder, but with violent suicide attempts [Neves et al. 2008]. So maybe this polymorphism is not exactly associated with the pathogenesis of bipolar disorder itself, but may lead to some symptoms shared with other psychiatric diseases. It may also cause certain personality traits that predispose for pathogenesis of bipolar disorder. The ss genotype leads for example to enhanced stress reactivity in general. A very recent study tested this 5-HTTLPR variant in relation to stress response in newborns. They tested the relation between genotype and cortisol release (a measurement for stress) after a foot prick, an element in a routine check, however, it was still associated with stress for the newborn. SS genotype carriers had much higher cortisol levels than other genotypes. Thus s-allele carriers show much higher stress response of the hypothalamus-pituitary-adrenal axis (HPA) than l-allele carriers [Müller et al. 2009]. Summarized serotonin transporter polymorphisms show inconclusive results; they seem to be involved in pathogenesis, but to a minor than expected.

3.4 Genes Involved in Biogenic Amine Modulation

3.4.1 MAOA

The antidepressant effect of monoamine oxidase inhibitors, the biochemical reaction of MAO in relationship with the monoaminergic neurotransmitter hypothesis of bipolar disorder, the relationship with clock genes, as well as some shared symptoms with Brunner's disease (mild mental retardation, impulsive-aggressive behavior, hypersexuality and attempted exhibitionism), which affects the chromosomal region of MAO, implicate a role of its gene variants in bipolar affective disorder [Bach et al. 1988; Brunner et al. 1993; Fiedorowicz et al. 2004]. The gene of monoamine-oxidase-A is located on chromosomal region Xp11.23-p11.4 and is expressed in the outer mitochondrial membrane. "Clock proteins" and other enhancers regulate the transcription of MAOA. Yet finally numerous other candidate genes for bipolar disorder can affect pathogenesis via monoamine oxidase [Hampp et al. 2008; Hampp and Albrecht 2008]. MAOA and MAOB degrade monoaminergic neurotransmitters and dietary amines by oxidative deamination of monoamines [Bach et al. 1988]. Oxygen is used to remove an amine group from a molecule, resulting in the corresponding aldehyde and ammonia. MAOA mainly breaks down 5-hydroxytryptamine (serotonin), norepinephrine (noradrenaline), and epinephrine (adrenaline), whereas MAOB prefers phenylethylamine. Both MAOs degrade dopamine [Shih et al. 2004].

Animal Studies

MAOA/B-double-knockout-mice have increased brain levels of serotonin, norepinephrine, dopamine, phenylethylamine and decreased serotonin metabolite 5-hydroxyindoleacetic acid levels [Cases et al. 1995; Chen et al. 2004]. MAOA-knockout-mice show aggressive behavior and have increased brain levels of serotonin (5-HT), norepinephrine (NE) and dopamine (DA) [Cases et al. 1995]. Also very rare human MAOA-null-allele-carriers show impulsive-aggressive behavior [Margit Burgmeister 2008]. MAOB deficient mice do not exhibit aggression, but have increased levels of the MAOB preferred substrate phenylethylamine [Shih et al. 2004].

Antidepressants

MAO inhibitors, which have been used since the 1950s [López-Muñoz F et al. 2007], have well studied antidepressant effects. These implicate MAO genes as candidate regions for affective disorders [Fiedorowicz et al. 2004].

Association Studies

Brunner discovered in 1993 a special point mutation, a 936C-T transition in the eighth exon of MAOA on chromosome X, which leads to mental retardation and behavioral problems including aggression, attempted rape, arson, exhibitionism and voyeurism. These impulsive, aggressive symptoms especially arouse during periods of 1-3 days with lack of sleep and are provoked by anger, often out of proportion to the provocation. Since manic-depressive illness comprises some elements of Brunner's disease (e.g. impulsive or dysphoric behavior, hypersexuality), this locus reached interest for association studies [Brunner et al. 1993].

CA-Repeat Microsatellite in Intron 2

The CA-repeat microsatellite polymorphism in intron 2, a well studied and promising polymorphism of MAOA [Black et al. 1991], was associated with bipolar disorder within Japanese and Caucasian population in a meta-analysis which pooled data from seven studies; namely from Furlong et al. 1999; Craddock et al., 1995, Lim et al., 1995, Parsian and Todd, 1997, Nöthen et al., 1995, Muramatsu et al., 1997, Kawada et al., 1995 [Furlong et al. 1999]. Additionally, other groups showed that some alleles of the microsatellite repeat polymorphism are significantly connected with bipolar affective disorder [Kawada et al. 1995; Lim et al. 1995; Rubinsztein et al. 1996]. Further meta-analysis, which included four association studies by Lim et al., Rubinsztein et al. Craddock et al., Parsian and Todd, proved association only for females [Preisig et al. 2000]. Nevertheless, some association studies as well as all recent GWAS failed to prove association [Nöthen et al., 1995; Parsian and Todd 1997; Muramatsu et al., 1997; Lin et al. 2008; Serretti et al. 2002; Baum et al. 2008, Wellcome Trust Consortium 2007; Sklar et al. 2008; Ferreira et al. 2008; Smith et al. 2009; Djurovic et al. 2010; Lee et al. 2011; Pereira et al. 2011; Belmonte et al. 2011; Cichon et al. 2011; Smith et al. 2011; Yosifova et al. 2011; Sklar et al. 2011; Chen et al. 2011; Kerner et al. 2011; Greenwood et al. 2012].

Fnu4H1 RFLP (Fnu4H1 Restriction Fragment Length Polymorphism)

The *Fnu4H1* RFLP polymorphism got its name due to an *Fnu4H1* site (a restriction enzyme cutting site), which is generated by a G to T substitution at the third base of codon 941 of MAOA. This substitution does not result in a change in amino acid at this position but is associated with increased activity of MAOA [Hotamisligil et al. 1991]. Recently Müller et al. investigated this MAOA polymorphism with the G to T substitution at position 941 and found marginal association for the T allele. Furthermore, he associated a special haplotype, comprising of this and other polymorphisms with manic-depressive illness [Müller et al. 2007]. Already in the late 1990s Rubinsztein and colleagues provided evidence of association for the Fnu4HI RFLP polymorphism and manic-depressive illness in a meta-analysis by combining their own results with British studies [Rubinsztein et al. 1996]. Also Furlong and colleagues proved association in a meta-analysis comprising seven studies [Furlong et al. 1999]. However, many studies could not prove any association with alleles of this MAOA sequence variance [Muramatsu et al., 1997; Preisig et al. 2000; Serretti et al. 2002].

EcoRV Polymorphism (T-to-C Substitution at Position–1460)

The sequence of this MAOA polymorphism resembles the restriction enzyme cutting site of *EcoRV* (a DNA endonuclease) and is produced by a T-to-C substitution at position –1460 [Hotamisligil et al. 1991]. A recent study by Huang showed that the MAOA sequence variance *EcoRV* was not associated with bipolar disorder [Huang et al. 2008].

T-to-A Substitution at Position 1077 (Promoter VNTR)

Another functional MAO polymorphism contains the MAOA gene-linked polymorphic region (MAOA-LPR) positioned approximately 1.2 kb upstream of the coding sequence. Five alleles of 2, 3, 3.5, 4, and 5 copies of the 30 bp repetitive sequence have been described. This polymorphism influences transcription activity of the MAO promoter [Sabol et al. 1998]. Nevertheless, there is significant evidence that this promoter polymorphism is not associated with manic-depressive disease since all studies rejected association with bipolar disorder [Furlong et al. 1999; Kunugi et al. 1999; Syagailo et al. 2001; Serretti et al. 2002; Müller et al. 2007; Huang et al. 2008; Lin et al. 2008].

Variable Number of Tandem Repeats (VNTR) Polymorphism in Intron 1

This VNTR (Variable Number of Tandem Repeats) polymorphism in intron 1 of MAOA is not associated with manic-depressive illness [Muramatsu et al. 1997; Preisig et al. 2000; Serretti et al. 2002].

Table 4: MAOA Polymorphisms and the Relationship with Bipolar Disorder (BD)

Polymorphism of MAO-A	Association with BD	No association with BD
CA-repeat microsatellite in intron 2	Kawada et al. 1995 Lim et al. 1995 Rubinsztein et al. 1996 Furlong et al. 1999 (meta-analysis) Preisig[1] et al. 2000	Nöthen et al.1995 Parsian and Todd 1997 Muramatsu et al. 1997 Serretti et al. 2002 Lin et al. 2008
Fnu4HI RFLP (MAOA–941T>G)	Rubinsztein et al. 1996 Furlong et al. 1999 Müller et al. 2007	Muramatsu et al. 1997 Preisig et al. 2000 Serretti et al. 2002
Polymorphic promoter VNTR polymorphism located ca. 1,200 bp upstream from the translation start site in the	Hu et al. 2013 (BD with comorbid alcoholisms in Chinese)	Furlong et al. 1999 Kunugi et al. 1999 Syagailo 2001

Polymorphism of MAO-A	Association with BD	No association with BD
MAOA-LPR (uVNTR polymorphism)		Serretti et al. 2002 Müller et al. 2007 Huang et al. 2008 Lin et al. 2008
VNTR polymorphism in intron 1		Muramatsu et al. 1997 Preisig et al. 2000 Serretti et al. 2002
EcoR polymorphism (–1460 T>C)		Serretti et al. 2002 Huang et al. 2008
1077 T>C		Serretti et al. 2002

1 for females

Linkage studies

X-linked heredity for bipolar disorder has been assumed for a long time, however, linkage analysis with X linked markers like G6PD deficiency, colorblindness, and factor IX had inconsistent results [Mendlewicz et al. 1973; Baron et al. 1987; Pekkarinen et al. 1995; Wigg et al. 2009]. MAOA and MAOB are closely linked in opposite orientation to the X chromosome at Xp11.23-p11.4 [Derry et al. 1989]. Some linkage studies discovered the chromosomal region of the MAOA gene in genome wide approaches [Zandi et al. 2001; Wigg et al. 2009; Pekkarinen et al. 1995].

3.4.2 MAOB

Two MAOB-association-studies investigated the relationship with bipolar disorder, but findings are negative. The dinucleotide repeat in the intron 2 (MAOB-GT) was not associated with bipolar affective disorder [Muramatsu et al. 1997; Parsian and Todd 1997].

3.4.3 COMT

The COMT gene is mapped to chromosomal region 22q11.1-q11.2. Catechol-O-methyltransferase (COMT) is a widely expressed enzyme, which inactivates catecholamines and catechol drugs such as L-DOPA. It catalyzes the transfer of a methyl group from S-adenosyl methionine to catecholamines, including the neurotransmitters dopamine, epinephrine and norepinephrine. This O-methylation results in one of the major degradative pathways of the catecholamine transmitters

[Hosak et al. 2007]. COMT polymorphisms confer significant genetic risk for psychiatric diseases, especially schizophrenia [Lewis et al. 2003; Shifman et al. 2004; Funke et al. 2005; Allen et al. 2008; Chien et al. 2009; Brisch et al. 2009; Hoenicka et al. 2010; Wang et al. 2009]. Not only schizophrenia is affected by COMT variants, but also bipolar disorder to a minor degree [Lachman 1996; Kirov 1998; Shifman 2004; Funke 2005; Goghari 2008; Zhang 2009]. A deletion on chromosome 22 (22q11), which leads to velocardiofacial syndrome, an autosomal dominant congenital disorder associated with cleft palate, cardiac defects and learning disabilities, helped to identify this causality. Due to common comorbidity of velocardiofacial syndrome with schizophrenia, bipolar disorder or attention deficit syndromes, this chromosomal region reached interest for genetic research [Carlson et al. 1997]. A polymorphism of the COMT gene, which leads to a valine-methionine substitution at amino acid 158 of the membrane-bound form of the enzyme, was found. This low activity polymorphism is associated with bipolar disorders in patients with velocardiofacial syndrome [Lachman et al. 1996]. Homozygosity for the COMT158met allele leads to a 3-4-fold reduction in enzymatic activity compared to homozygotes for the COMT158val allele. There is also a good chance that the low activity allele is associated with bipolar disorder [Lachman et al. 1996]. In general this COMT polymorphism was often associated with bipolar disorder by many association studies [Lachman et al. 1996; Kirov et al. 1998; Shifman et al. 2004; Funke et al, 2005; Goghari et al. 2008]. A recent large Chinese study, comprising of 478 BP patients and 469 healthy subjects, showed significant association between the Val/Met polymorphism and bipolar disorder. They also conducted a meta-analysis on 19 studies and reached significant positive results for the Met allele of the polymorphism [Zhang et al. 2009]. Although there have been many positive results, some other studies suggested no association [Gutierrez et al. 1997, Kirov et al. 1999; Kunugi et al. 1997; Geller et al. 2000]. This polymorphism was also investigated for rapid cycling and ultra-ultra rapid cycling in young patients with positive [Kirov et al. 1998; Papolos et al. 1998] and negative results [Geller et al. 2000]. Nevertheless, Kirov and colleagues showed association of the Met allele with rapid cycling [Kirov et al. 1998]. Epigenetic changes influence also COMT expression and the risk of bipolar disorder. Hypomethylation of the COMT promoter leads to increased risk for bipolar disorder and schizophrenia. Thus also epigenetic changes should be considered. Maybe they are the missing part of the puzzle within inconsistent research results [Abdolmaleky et al. 2006].

Table 5: COMT Gene Variants and Association with Bipolar Disorder (BD)

COMT polymorphism	Association with BD	No association with BD
Val/Met polymorphism (rs4680; Met-allele is the low-activity allele)	Lachman et al. 1996 Kirov et al. 1998 Shifman et al. 2004 Funke et al. 2005 Goghari et al. 2008 Zhang et al. 2009 (large study and meta-analys on 19studies) Lee et al. 2010 Benedetti et al. 2011 Nohesara et al. 2011 (epigenetic study)	Gutierrez et al. 1997 Kunugi et al. 1997 Kirov et al. 1999 Geller et al. 2000

3.4.4 TPH

TPH, which codes for Tryptophan hydroxylase, maps to the chromosomal region 11p15.3-p14 [Nielsen et al. 1992]. Tryptophan hydroxylase (TPH) is the rate limiting and first enzyme of serotonin synthesis. TPH initiates serotonin synthesis by hydroxylation of tryptophan, which results in 5-hydroxytryptophan. Then an aromatic-amino-acid-decarboxylase produces serotonin. Since TPH is the first and rate-limiting enzyme in serotonin synthesis its gene has been suggested to be involved in affective disorders. TPH1, expressed in peripheral tissues [Walther et al. 2003], shows no evidence of association with bipolar disorder [Vincent et al. 1999; Lai et al. 2005; Choi et al. 2010], yet it might influence suicidality [Galfalvy et al. 2009]. TPH2 is a recently discovered isoform encoded on chromosome 12, which is expressed predominantly in serotonergic neurons in the brain [Walther et al. 2003; Zhang et al. 2004]. The -C8347G promoter SNP (rs4131347), which leads to a cytosine to guanine exchange at position 8347, seems not to be associated with mood disorder [Mann et al. 2008]. Also the A218C polymorphism of TPH was not associated with bipolar disorder [Rietschel et al. 2000]. However, significant haplotype association of TPH2 polymorphisms and BD were identified in two recent association studies [Lopez et al. 2007; Lin et al. 2007]. Recently Cichon and colleagues also showed significant association with bipolar disorder for the TPH 2 variants rs11178997 and rs17110563 (leading to a Pro206Ser substitution) in a sample of a total of 883 patients and 1300 controls from Germany and Russia, which included two cohorts of bipolar disorder. Interestingly the TPH2 Pro206Ser mutation leads to reduced thermal stability and solubility of the enzyme TPH2 and leads to reduced serotonin production in the brain. The association between the Pro206Ser variant and bipolar disorder was later replicated in 198 bipolar patients and 180 controls in a Romanian sample [Cichon et al. 2008; Grigoroiu-Serbanescu et al. 2010]. Furthermore, TPH seems to play a role in suicidal behavior [Tsai et al. 1999; Campos et al. 2010]. Contrastively, one small study of the late 90s suggested no association with suicide [Furlong et al. 1997]. Serretti and colleagues investigated also the relationship between major psychosis and the TPH A218C gene variant in a large pedigree (1424 patients in total; 627 patients with bipolar disorder, 511 patients with major depressive disorder, 210 patients with schizophrenia, 48 with delusional disorder and 27 patients with psychotic disorder not otherwise specified). Yet, they did not find significant association with major psychosis but a trend towards association with bipolar disorder [Serretti et al. 2001]. Furthermore, TPH2 polymorphisms were associated with bipolar disorder and comorbid panic disorder in 515 patients (274 patients with BD (subtypes I and II), including 45 patients with lifetime panic disorder comorbidity and 241 controls) [Campos et al. 2011]. Polymorphisms of TPH and serotonin transporter seem to influence the response to SSRI and could be future markers for treatment decisions [Serretti et al. 2001; Serretti et al. 2004]. Recently Serretti and colleagues disproved this relationship between treatment response and TPH polymorphisms in a very small and inhomogenous sample (145 patients with major depression, 132 patients with bipolar disorder, 221 patients with schizophrenia and 170 psychiatrically healthy controls) [Serretti et al. 2011]. Although TPH1 and TPH2, as well as genes involved in the serotonergic system in general, did not belong to top hits of GWAS, the serotonergic metabolism still seems to have an important role in affective disorders to a minor degree [Baum et al. 2008; Wellcome Trust Consortium 2007; Sklar 2008; Ferreira 2008; Smith et al. 2009; Djurovic et al. 2010; Lee et al. 2011; Pereira et al. 2011; Belmonte et al. 2011; Cichon et al. 2011; Smith et al. 2011; Yosifova et al. 2011; Sklar et al. 2011; Chen et al. 2011; Kerner et al. 2011; Greenwood et al. 2012].

3.4.5 TH

Tyrosin hydroxylase (TH) is encoded on 11p15 and is responsible for the first step in the synthesis of catecholamines by converting tyrosine into L-dopa. TH and TPH, the biosynthetic enzymes for norepinephrine and 5-HT, were reduced in the locus coeruleus of bipolar suicide victims, which lead to an imbalance of norepinephrine and serotonin. So TH and TPH seem to be involved in pathogenesis of mood disorders [Wiste et al. 2008]. Also linkage studies supposed a relationship between the tyrosine hydroxylase locus and mood disorders [Malfosse et al. 1997; Smyth et al. 1997; Craddock et al. 1999; Serretti et al. 2000]. The microsatellite polymorphism HUMTH01 of TH is characterized by a TCAT repeat motif. In an analysis and meta-analysis by Furlong this polymorphism was not associated with unipolar or bipolar disorder [Furlong et al. 1999]. A large multicenter case-control association study, comprising 401 bipolar patients and 401 controls, investigated the tetranucleotide polymorphism of TH and could not find evidence of association with manic depressive disease either [Souery et al. 1999], but TH was significantly associated in association studies of major depressive disorder. Although results of linkage studies of bipolar disorder were promising association studies and GWAS did not show hints of involvement with bipolar disorder [Serretti et al. 1998; Baum et al. 2008; Wellcome Trust Consortium 2007; Sklar et al. 2008, Ferreira 2008; Smith et al. 2009; Djurovic et al. 2010; Lee et al. 2011; Pereira et al. 2011; Belmonte et al. 2011; Cichon et al. 2011; Smith et al. 2011; Yosifova et al. 2011; Sklar et al. 2011; Chen et al. 2011; Kerner et al. 2011; Greenwood et al. 2012].

3.5 Clock Genes

Many processes in organism (including release of melatonin or cortisone, body temperature) underlie circadian rhythm operated by an endogen clock. A specialized and centralized pace maker in CNS as well as in peripheral organs and tissues was found. Seasonal changes of mood, sleep disturbance in affective disorders as well as antidepressant effects of light therapy and sleep deprivation indicate a role of the circadian system in the pathogenesis of mood disorders [Lee et al. 2007; McClung 2007]. Also Lithium, a powerful mood stabilizer, modulates circadian rhythms via inhibition of glycogen-synthase-kinase-3-beta (GSK3B) and thus suggests a role of clock genes in bipolar disorder [Yin et al. 2006].

3.5.1 The Circadian Oscillator in the Suprachiasmatic Nucleus

Circadian rhythms are generated in the suprachiasmatic nucleus (SCN) and connected peripheral oscillators [Moore 1999]. The SCN is located in the anterior hypothalamus above the optic chiasm and its core is linked to light/dark cycles by a direct retinal innervation, the retinohypothalamic tract [Abrahamson et al. 2001]. So light at dusk or dawn can help the SCN to function in an exact 24 hour rhythm by starting gene expression albeit the SCN can also maintain almost circadian rhythms without any cues from environment [Porterfield et al. 2009]. Therefore the SCN can help to adapt physiological and hormonal rhythms to the environmental light-dark cycle. Many physiological processes, for example wakefulness, sleep, mood, food intake, metabolisms, hormonal and cardiovascular rhythms are dependent on circadian rhythms. Beside the SCN can also recognize seasonal changes by measuring the lengths of a day. Also food-intake and other information like temperature can synchronize the clock [Mendoza 2006]. The 24-hour rhythms are regulated by an intrinsic circadian oscillator located in the SCN and based on interlinked auto regulatory positive and negative transcriptional/ translational feedback loops [Shearman et al. 2000; Cermakian et al. 2003].

Course of action: 1. The cycle begins with heterodimerization of Arntl (Bmal1 or Mop3) and Clock [Gekakis et al. 1998] (or alternatively Npas can bind Arntl (Bmal1) [DeBruyne et al. 2007]). 2. The Arntl-Clock heterodimer binds to e-box enhancers (transcription factor binding sites) of several clock genes, including PER (period genes) and CRY (Cryptochrome genes) and activates their transcription [Gekakis et al. 1998; Langmesser et al. 2008]. 3. Per and Cry proteins accumulate after 12hours in the cytoplasm and get phosphorylated by two casein kinases Csnk1, Csnk1E or glycogen-synthase-kinase-3b (Gsk3B). The phosphorylation of PER genes modulates the length of the cycle [Etchegaray et al.2009]. Then, phosphorylated Per and Cry proteins form heterodimers and enter the nucleus. There the Per and Cry protein complexes suppress their own transcription by binding the Arntl-Clock heterodimers and therefore creating a negative feedback loop [Langmesser et al. 2008]. In addition Clock/Bmal1 complexes initiate transcription of retinoic acid-related orphan nuclear receptors (REV-ERBa and RORa) genes. The gene products, Rev-erba and RORa, can bind to ROREs (retinoic acid-related orphan receptor response elements) in the promoter of ARNTL (BMAL1) and can therefore regulate the expression of BMAL1. RORs activate, whereas REV-ERBa inhibit the transcription of BMAL1 [Raspé et al. 2002].

Table 6: Function of Clock genes

Clock gene	Function of Clock gene
CLOCK	A dimer of Clock and Arntl is the main transcriptional activator of many clock genes (including CRY1 and 2 and PER 1-3 genes). Clock and Arntl activate transcription of REV-ERBa gene (NR1D1). Clock activates transcription of Dbp, another clock gene product
ARNTL (BMAL1 or MOP3)	Arntl heterodimers with Npas2 bind to promoter e-boxes of MAOA. This leads to transcription of MAOA and finally to inactivation of dopamine and inhibition of the promanic effect of dopamine! Arntl also activates the transcription of other clock genes (PER1, PER2, PER3, and CRY1, CRY2).
NPAS2	
PER1	Per proteins associate with Cry1 and Cry2. Phosphorylated Cry and Per protein complexes enter the nucleus and suppress their own transcription by binding Arntl-Npas2 or Arntl-Clock heterodimers (negative feedback loop).
PER2	
PER3	
CRY1	CRY genes code for cryptochromes, which are mammalian circadian photoreceptors in the retina and pacemaker elements in the SCN
CRY2	
CSNK1d	Casein kinase 1 delta and Casein kinase 1 epsilon phosphorylate core genes of the circadian oscillator (Per1, Per2, Per3 and Cry1, Cry2, Cry3). Phosphorylation of PER genes is a speed-determining step in the circadian cycle and modulates cycle length.
CSNK1e	
NRIDI (REV-ERBa)	Inhibits transcription of ARNTL (BMAL1). Inhibits Clock and Npas2. Major regulator of cyclic ARNTL transcription. Lithium leads to degradation of NRIDI (REV-ERBa gene)
PPARGCIB	This clock protein may bind to RORE sites of ARNTL and NR1D1 and influences their transcription
THRA	Important thyroid nuclear receptor gene
DBP	Dbp controls expression of many clock genes
TIMELESS	"Clock protein", which is regulated by CLOCK and ARNTL
BHLHB2	Basic helix-loop-helix transcription factor, which represses the Clock/Bmal1-induced transactivation of the Per1 promoter through direct protein-protein interactions with Bmal1 and/or competition for E-box elements.

3.5.2 Role of clock genes in bipolar disorder

ARNTL (BMAL1 or MOP3)

Many candidate genes for bipolar disorder code for elements of the previous described intrinsic circadian oscillator. ARNTL (BMAL1 or MOP3), a top candidate in functional analysis of GWAS data, is a key element of the molecular circadian oscillator [Le-Niculescu et al. 2008; Nievergelt et al. 2009; Bunger et al. 2000]. ARNTL (BMAL1) is very important for the final effect of the circa dian feedback loop, which leads to transcription of clock genes (CRY1 and 2 and PER 1, PER2, PER3) and the dopamine degrading enzyme MAOA. Arntl and Npas2 build heterodimers and bind e-boxes of the MAOA promoter. This leads to transcription and protein synthesis of MAOA. Thus dopamine gets degraded and the promanic effect of dopamine vanishes [Hampp et al. 2008; Hampp and Albrecht 2008; Kripke et al. 2009]. ARNTL (BMAL1) knockout mice have disrupted circadian rhythms and show decreased activity [McDearmon et al. 2006]. Many association studies have already proven a connection between individual SNPs (Single Nucleotide Polymorphisms) of ARNTL and bipolar affective disorder [Mansour et al. 2006; Nievergelt et al. 2006; Le-Niculescu et al. 2008; Mansour et al. 2009], while others could not replicate this finding recently [Kripke et al. 2009; Shi et al. 2008]. Also special haplotypes in ARNTL and PER3 are significantly associated with bipolar disorder [Nievergelt et al. 2006].

NPAS2

Npas2 is an important clock protein encoded on 2q13, which initiates the transcription of many clock genes together with Arntl (Bmal1). The NPAS2 SNP rs1562313 has been associated with bipolar disorder recently as well as rs13025524 and rs11123857 [Kripke et al. 2009; Mansour et al. 2009]. Besides NPAS2 may also have a role in seasonal affective disorder [Johannson et al. 2003]. Yet those findings could not be proven by Nievergelt and colleagues [Nievergelt et al. 2006].

NR1D1

NR1D1 (Nuclear Receptor REV-ERBa Gene), another candidate gene for bipolar disorder, is located on chromosome 17. NR1D1 inhibits on one hand the transcription of ARNTL by inhibitory binding to ARNTL RORE promoter sites and on the other hand the activation of ARNTL by Clock and Npas2. This leads to decreased MAOA effects and higher promanic dopamine levels. Some gene variants of NR1D1 e.g. rs2314339 and special haplotypes are strongly associated with bipolar disorder [Kripke et al. 2009; Severino et al. 2009]. Nuclear Receptor Rev-erba is also a critical Lithium-sensitive component and may support the pathogenesis of manic-depressive disorder [Yin et al. 2006]. So NR1D1 seems to be a promising candidate gene even though Shi and colleagues could not prove this association [Shi et al. 2008].

Period Genes (PER1, PER2, PER3)

Some PER3 SNPs and certain haplotypes have been associated with bipolar disorder in family-based and case-control association studies [Nievergelt et al. 2006; Mansour et al. 2006]. Nievergelt and colleagues found the strongest association with a certain haplotype, which included a combination of 6 markers of PER3 (four intronic markers rs228729, rs228642, rs228666, and rs2859388, a non-synonymous SNP in exon 17 (rs228697) and the 54-bp length polymorphism in exon 18). Beside this haplotype other combinations of PER3 gene markers also showed modest association. Some haplotypes of PER3 may have a protective effect, for instance a haplotype comprising of two intronic SNPs (rs3789327 and rs2278749) lead to resilience [Nievergelt et al. 2006]. Furthermore, certain length variants of PER3 with variable-number-tandem-repeat (VNTR) polymorphism influence age of onset. Homozygotes of this PER3 length variant progress bipolar disorder at young age [Benedetti et al. 2006]. While many studies support association of PER3 polymorphisms with bipolar disorder, Kripke et al. could not replicate these findings in a recent association study [Kripke et al. 2009]. At least polymorphisms of PER3 were observed in delayed sleep-phase syndrome and sleep dysregulation in mood disorders indicating a role in symptoms, which are very common in mood disorders [Pereira et al. 2005; Archer et al. 2003; Ebisawa et al. 2001].

PER2, another clock gene, is a further candidate for bipolar disorder. Kripke and colleagues showed modest evidence of association for three SNPs (Single Nucleotide Polymorphisms) of PER2 (rs4663868, rs2304672 and rs2304669) [Kripke et al. 2009]. Per2 might have an impact on mood via transcription of MAOA, because it can regulate transcription of the enzyme either. A certain mutation of PER2 in mice leads to decreased expression of MAOA and thus increased dopamine levels and promanic behavior. Mice mutants of PER2 also show changed behavior towards cocaine response, increased alcohol consumption and lack of food anticipation [Hampp et al. 2008]. Furthermore, PER2 has been associated with advanced sleep syndrome [Toh et al. 2001]. Finally, a PER2 polymorphism in the binding site of the clock protein CKIe in PER2 was not associated with bipolar disorder [Shiino et al. 2003].

CRY

CRY1 located on 12q23-q24.1 lies within a hot spot discovered in multiple linkage studies and even in genome wide approaches for bipolar disorder [Ewald et al. 2002; Glaser et al. 2005, Green et al. 2005; Cassidy et al. 2007]. This region is closely linked to Darier's disease, which shows association with bipolar disorder [Green et al. 2005]. Although this region is strongly linked to bipolar disorder, association studies could not prove a connection of CRY1 to bipolar disorder, as well as to the second cryptochrome gene CRY2 on chromosomal region 11p11.2 [Nievergelt et al. 2005; Mansour et al. 2006; Nievergelt et al. 2006; Shi et al. 2008]. Meanwhile, others showed nominal association [Mansour et al. 2009].

CLOCK

CLOCK is located on chromosomal region 4q12 and codes for a basic helix-loop-helix (bHLH)-PAS transcription factor for several clock genes [King et al. 1997]. Many animal studies and association studies indicated a role in mood disorders. Disruption of CLOCK leads to manic-like behavior in mice [Roybal et al. 2007]. Kripke and colleagues supported evidence of association for many SNPs of CLOCK with bipolar disorder in a recent association study [Kripke et al. 2009]. Also Shi et al. found modest evidence of association with bipolar disorder for several individual SNPs (e.g. rs534654, rs6850524 and rs4340844) and haplotypes of CLOCK. An interaction of 3 SNPs in the CLOCK gene region, the BHLHB2 gene and CSNK1E, was significantly associated with bipolar disorder [Shi et al. 2008]. On the other hand Kishi et al. could not find significant association of CLOCK with bipolar disorder in the Japanese population; neither could Mansour et al. and Nievergelt et al. in Caucasian pedigree [Kishi et al. 2009; Mansour et al. 2006; Nievergelt et al. 2006]. A CLOCK variant (T3111C polymorphism = rs1801260) at the 3' untranslated region of CLOCK is involved in a high recurrence rate of bipolar disorder [Benedetti et al. 2003], as well as in sleep dysregulation in bipolar patients [Serretti et al. 2007]. The T3111C polymorphism was also investigated for association with major depression, but Desan et al. could not find any correlation [Desan et al. 2000]. Nevertheless, CLOCK is a very important gene in circadian regulation and therefore a candidate gene for mood disorders.

DBP

DBP codes for a D-box binding protein and is located on chromosome 19. Animal studies suggested a role of DBP in bipolar disorder. Total DBP-knockout-mice produce bipolar behavior [Niculescu et al. 2000; Le-Niculescu et al. 2008]. Nonetheless, results of association studies were rather disappointing [Nievergelt et al. 2006; Shi et al. 2008].

CSNKD

The region of the CSNKD gene on chromosome 17 was significantly linked to bipolar disorder in an early genome wide approach [Dick et al. 2003]. Kripke et al. found an association of the CSNK1D SNP rs4510078 with bipolar disorder recently [Kripke et al.2009]; however, it could not be replicated by Shi et al. [Shi et al. 2008].

CSNKE

Casein-kinase-1-delta and Casein-kinase-1-epsilon phosphorylate core genes of the circadian oscillator (PER1, PER2, PER3 and CRY1, CRY2, CRY3). Phosphorylation of Per is a speed determining step in the circadian cycle and modulates cycle length. Some gene variants for those casein kinases were linked with manic-depressive illness in linkage studies [Nievergelt et al. 2006]. Shi et al. found that a multi-locus interaction between rs6442925 in the 5' upstream of BHLHB2, rs1534891 in CSNK1E, and rs534654 near the 3' end of the CLOCK gene is significantly associated with manic depressive disorder [Shi et al. 2008].

TIMELESS

TIMELESS is located in the chromosomal region 12q12-q13 and its transcription is regulated by Clock and Bmal1. Mansour et al. observed modest association of some TIMELESS single-nucleotide-polymorphisms and manic-depressive-disorder [Mansour et al. 2006].

PPARGC1B

The PPARGC1B coding SNP, rs7732671 (Pro203Ala), might be associated with unipolar and bipolar affective disorder. This clock protein may bind to RORE sites of Arntl and NR1D1 and influence their transcription [Kripke et al. 2009].

Summary of clock genes

Table 7: All Clock Genes and Their Association with Bipolar Disorder (BD)

Clock gene	Chromosomal region	Support of association with bipolar disorder	No support of association with bipolar disorder
DBP	19q13.3	Niculescu et al. 2000	Shi et al. 2008
PER1	17p13.1-17p12	Kripke et al. 2009	Mansour et al. 2006 Nievergelt et al. 2006 Shi et al. 2008
PER2	2q37.3	Kripke et al. 2009	Shiino et al. 2003 Mansour et al. 2006 Nievergelt et al. 2006 Shi et al. 2008
PER3	1p36.23	Nievergelt et al. 2006 Mansour et al. 2006 Benedetti et al. 2008	Shi et al. 2008 Kripke et al. 2009
ARNTL (BMAL1 or MOP3)	11p15	Mansour et al. 2006 Nievergelt et al. 2006 Le-Niculescu et al. 2008	Shi et al. 2008 Kripke et al. 2009
ARNTL2	12p12.2-p11.2		Shi et al. 2008
NPAS2	2q13	Kripke et al. 2009	Nievergelt et al. 2006
CRY1	12q23-q24.1	Ewald et al. 2002 Glaser et al. 2005 Green et al. 2005 Cassidy et al. 2007	Nievergelt et al. 2005 Mansour et al. 2006 Shi et al. 2008
CRY2	11p11.2		Mansour et al. 2006 Nievergelt et al. 2006
CSNK1D	17q25		Shi et al. 2008
NRIDI (REV-ERBa)	17q11.2	Kripke et al. 2009 Severino et al. 2009	Shi et al. 2008
CLOCK	4q12	Shi et al. 2008 Kripke et al. 2009	Mansour et al. 2006 Nievergelt et al. 2006 Kishi et al. 2009
THRA	17q11.2	Kripke et al. 2009	
CSNKID		Kripke et al. 2009	
TIMELESS	12q12-q13	Mansour et al. 2006	Shi et al. 2008
CSNK1ε	22q13.1	Nievergelt et al. 2006 Shi et al. 2008	
BHLHB2	3p26	Shi et al. 2008	

3.6 Growth Hormones

3.6.1 BDNF

Functions of BDNF

The BDNF gene is a highly controversial but important candidate gene in bipolar disorder. It is coded in the chromosomal region 11p13-15 [Egeland et al. 1987; Schumacher et al. 2005]. Bdnf is a member of the neurotrophin superfamily and is the most abundant and distributed neurotrophic factor in the brain [Sklar et al. 2002]. It has several important functions like neuronal survival [Kirschenbaum et al. 1995], migration, myelination, phenotypic differentiation, neurogenesis [Zigova et al. 1998; Pencea et al. 2001], axonal, and dendritic growth and synapse formation [Keri Martinowich 2008]. Additionally it has an important role in neural plasticity and behavior. BDNF expression is also very important for learning and memory; it has antidepressant effects and leads to serotonergic axon growth and sprouting [Binder et al. 2004; Rybakowski 2009; Mamounas et al. 1995].

Table 8: Functions of Bdnf (Brain Derived Neurotrophic Factor)

Functions of Bdnf	
– Neuronal migration – Neuronal regeneration – Phenotypic differentiation – Serotonergic axon growth – Synapse formation – Myelination	– Neuronal survival and growth – Key regulator of synaptic plasticity – Memory acquisition and consolidation – Antidepressant effect

BDNF Signal Transduction

The various functions of BDNF are mediated by two receptor systems TrkB and p75NTR. Binding of mature Bdnf to TrkB leads to tyrosine phosphorylation in its cytoplasmic domain that finally activates the MEK–MAPK, phosphatidylinositol-3-kinase (PI-3-K) and phospholipase C-g (PLC-g) signaling pathways. The signal transduction via TrkB regulates most functions of Bdnf. Binding of the proneurotrophin to p75NTR ends in activation of apoptotic signaling and NMDA receptor-dependent synaptic depression in the hippocampus [Martinowich et al. 2008; Binder et al. 2004].

BDNF Polymorphisms

Dinucleotide repeat (GT)n (BDNF-LCPR)

An intronic microsatellite (GT)n dinucleotide repeat marker at position -1040 of the BDNF gene might be associatiated with mood disorder [Neves-Pereira et al. 2002; Strauss et al. 2004].

Val66Met Polymorphism

A single nucleotide polymorphism (SNP) of BDNF, which carries an exchange of the 66th amino acid valine into methionine (Val66Met) in the pro-domain of BDNF, leads to problems in trafficking of the neurotrophin [Rybakowski et al. 2008]. The amino acid change is based on a G/A substitution at nucleotide 196, for this reason this polymorphism is also called G196A [De Luca et al. 2008]. Val66Met carriers show deficits in short-term episodic memory and show abnormal hippocampal morphology [Pezawas et al. 2004; Rybakowski et al. 2008]. The frequency of Val or Met allele shows ethnic differences [Rybakowski et al. 2008; Petryshen et al. 2009]. This polymorphism seems to affect many psychiatric disease and neurodegenerative disorders including Parkinson's and Alzheimer's disease. Even an association between Bdnf function and epilepsy was suggested. Beside Bdnf has also impact on pain transduction [Binder et al.2004]. Lately this polymorphism was often associated with bipolar disorder [Hashimoto et al. 2004]. The rare Met allele (=A-allele) of the Val66Met polymorphism also correlates with lower overall neuroticism scores [Sklar et al. 2009]

Association of BDNF Variants with Bipolar Disorder

Antidepressants, Mood Stabilizers and Animal Studies

Depressive states in rats show a decrement in levels of Bdnf in the hippocampus [Nibuya et.al.1995; Smith et al. 1995]. Further evidence for involvement of BDNF in affective disorders is the fact that antidepressants, electroconvulsive therapy and mood stabilizers raise BDNF expression in the brain [Duman et al. 1998; Chang et al. 2009]. Rat studies also showed that BDNF leads to growth of serotonin neurons in the brain [Mamounas 1999]. Bdnf even has antidepressant effects by itself if admitted directly into the brain of animal models [Rybakowski 2009].

Serum Levels of BDNF

Bdnf levels are abnormally reduced in manic and depressed states of bipolar disorder. This is proven by a meta-analysis and several studies [Cunha et al. 2006; Matute et al. 2006; Lin et al. 2009; de Oliveira et al. 2009; Tramontina et al. 2009]. Kauer-Sant'Anna claimed that only late stage bipolar disorder shows decreased Bdnf serum levels [Kauer-Sant'Anna et al. 2009]. Monteleone and colleagues discovered that Bdnf is even decreased in euthymic phases of bipolar and unipolar disorder independent from treatment [Monteleone et al. 2008]. Thus Bdnf may be a marker for bipolar disorder. Bdnf levels are also decreased in transformed lymphoblasts of patients treated with Lithium [Tseng et al. 2008], although results are inconsistent whether levels are still decreased after treatment [Tramontina et al. 2009]. Bdnf serum levels may also be a tool to differ between major depression and depressive episodes during bipolar disorder; patients with major depression have higher serum levels than depressed bipolar patients [Fernandes et al. 2009]. However, some studies show lowered Bdnf levels in unipolar depression as well [Monteleone et al. 2008].

Linkage studies for chromosome 11

Early linkage studies assumed linkage of bipolar disorder to the chromosomal region 11p15. Egeland and colleagues reported the first evidence for linkage to this region, which codes for BDNF, in Old Order Amish people [Egeland et.al. 1987]. Yet, reanalysis of a larger pedigree of Amish people revoked no linkage of bipolar disorder to chromosome 11 [Pauls et al. 1991]. Genome wide linkage studies found association of the following loci 11p15, 11p13-q13 on the 11th chromosome [Schumacher et al. 2005].

GWAS- Genome wide association studies

Early genome wide scans detected the chromosomal region 11p13–p14 as a locus of high interest [McInnes et al. 1996]. Le-Niculescu and colleagues discovered BDNF as one of the top candidate genes for bipolar disorder. Beside BDNF also other growth factor genes and growth factor receptor genes like NRG1, FGF12 and PTN were associated with bipolar disorder in a large GWAS [Le-Niculescu et al. 2009] while other recent genome wide association studies could not find any association of SNPs with bipolar disorder [Baum et al. 2008; Wellcome Trust Consortium 2007; Sklar et al. 2008, Ferreira et al. 2008; Smith et al. 2009; Djurovic et al. 2010; Lee et al. 2011, Pereira et al. 2011; Belmonte et al. 2011; Cichon et al. 2011; Smith et al. 2011; Yosifova et al. 2011; Sklar et al. 2011; Chen et al. 2011; Kerner et al. 2011; Greenwood et al. 2012].

Genetic association studies and family based genetic studies

Many studies claim significant association between BDNF gene variants, especially the Val66Met polymorphism, and bipolar disorder [Neves-Pereira et al. 2002; Sklar et al. 2002; Geller et al. 2004; Lohoff et al. 2005; Green et al. 2006; Müller et al.2006; Vincze et al. 2008; Xu et al. 2009; Liu et al. 2008; DeLuca et al.2008; Fan and Sklar 2008; Xu et al. 2009; Xu et al. 2010], while many others cannot find any association at all [Nakata et al. 2003; Hong et al. 2003; Skibinska 2004; Kunugi et al. 2004; Oswald et al. 2004; Kanazawa et al. 2007; Kim et al. 2008; Mick et al.2009]. Two groups could not find significant association with bipolar disorder in general, but with the subtype rapid cycling [Green et al. 2006; Müller et al. 2006]. Besides an interaction between the Val66Met polymorphism and the short allele of the 5HTTLPR, polymorphism of the serotonin transporter was reported in animal models of bipolar disorder. However, this interaction could not be proven in humans, although both variants confered risk to bipolar disorder in this study [Vincze et al. 2008]. BDNF was, nevertheless, identified as a top candidate in a functional analysis of large genome wide association studies, so involvement of this gene should be considered in pathogenesis [Le-Niculescu et al. 2009].

Reasons for controversies

One reason for the contrary study results might be the considerable diversity of BDNF polymorphisms among worldwide populations [Petryshen et al. 2009]. Most negative findings were done in Asian populations, where allele frequencies differ significantly to Europeans. Limited statistic power is another possibility for diverging results in different studies. Larger sample sizes of thousands are necessary for studies of genes with small effect. Inhomogeneity of the study population might be another factor for contrary results. It may not be a good idea to mix patients with bipolar I, bipolar II, and schizoaffective disorders, as it is done in some studies [Lohoff et al. 2005].

BDNF and subtypes of bipolar disorder or related disease

Rapid cycling

Another reason for inconsistent findings might be that some BDNF gene polymorphisms are only linked to some subtypes of bipolar disorder, for instance rapid cycling. Green et al. carried out a case-control study with over 3000 individuals from UK and could not find evidence for the association of the Val66Met polymorphism of BDNF with bipolar disorder, but they found significant association of the common Val allele with rapid cycling [Green et al. 2006]. They used the DSM-IV definition of rapid cycling, which needs 4 or more distinct episodes of major affective disorder within a 12 month period; such that consecutive distinct episodes are either switches of pole or are separated by at least 2 months of euthymia [Green et al. 2006; Müller et al. 2006]

Early onset bipolar disorder

Early onset bipolar disorder is more severe and related with an early onset in childhood. Geller et al. reported significant association of the BDNF Val66 allele to preadolescent bipolar disorder [Geller et al. 2004]. Mick et al. tried to replicate this finding, but failed. They could not prove any association to this Val66 allele, which carries an amino acid substitution (valine to methionine) at codon 66 of the BDNF gene [Mick et al. 2009]. Strauss et al. showed association of another BDNF variant, the 168 bp allele of the BDNF (GT)n dinucleotide repeat, with childhood-onset mood disorder [Strauss et al. 2004].

Suicidal behavior and BDNF

The Val/Met polymorphism of the BDNF gene might also lead to suicidal behavior. Patients with the Met/Met phenotype of the Val66Met polymorphism of the BDNF gene have an almost 5 times higher rate of suicide attempts. Maybe one day BDNF levels will be biological indicators for risk of suicide [Kim et al. 2008]. Again, findings are inconsistent. Some studies claim no association of suicidal behavior to BDNF Val66Met polymorphism [Hong et al. 2003].

Summary of Association Studies for BDNF and Bipolar Disorder (BD)

Table 9: BDNF Association Studies For Bipolar Disorder

Association of BDNF SNPs with BD	No association of BDNF SNPs with BD
Sklar et al. 2002: Val allele of the Val66Met polymorphism of BDNF is associated with BP in 470 parent-proband trios. Neves-Pereira et al. 2002: Association of the (GT)n-repeat and the G-allele of theVal66Met polymorphism with BD in a sample of 283 Caucasian nuclear families. Geller et al. 2004: 53 complete, independent trios (bipolar child and parents). Association of the Val allele of Val66Met polymorphism with prepubertal bipolar disorder. Lohoff et al. 2005: This study (621 Caucasian bipolar patients and 998 controls) showed association of the Val allele (of the val66met polymorphism) with bipolar disorder. Green et al. 2006: British case control sample of 3062 participants. Val allele is associated with rapid cycling. Müller et al.2006: Family-association study with 312 nuclear families showed association of BDNF variants with rapid cycling. Vincze et al. 2008: Association with the val66met polymorphism in a study of 447 Caucasian BD patients and 370 controls. Liu et al. 2008: 1749 Caucasian probands in 250 multiplex bipolar families. Many SNPs of BDNF are associated DeLuca et al.2008: Family-based association study in 312 BD Caucasian nuclear families showed association of BDNF Val66 to BD. Fan and Sklar 2008: Meta-analysis of all original published association studies up to May 2007. 14studies consisting of 4248cases and 7080controls and 858 nuclear families show modest, but significant evidence for association of Val66Met polymorphism with BD. Xu et al. 2009: Association with Val66Met polymorphism in Han Chinese. Chinese association study of 498 bipolar cases and 501 controls. Association of Val66Met polymorphism with BD.	Nakata et al. 2003: Matched case-control association design in a Japanese population (with 190 controls and 132 bipolar patients) shows no association with the two polymorphisms (21360C ->T and 196G-> A) and bipolar disorder. Hong et al. 2003: Chinese sample, 192 patients (84 MD and 108 BD) and 293 healthy controls. No association of Val66Met with bipolar disorder. Skibinska 2004: Val66Met of BDNF gene was studied in 336schizophrenics, 352 patients with BD and 375 healthy controls. Kunugi et al. 2004: A multi-center study of 519 Japanese patients with bipolar disorder and 588 controls claims that the Val66Met polymorphism is unrelated to bipolar disorder. Oswald et al. 2004: Association study with 112 bipolar patients and 163 controls. No association of Val66Met polymorphism and bipolar disorder. Kanazawa et al. 2007: Meta-analysis of 11 case-control studies (with 3143 patients with bipolar disorder and 6347 controls) showed no association of Val66Met polymorphism with BD Kim et al. 2008: Study with 169 bipolar Korean patients and 251 controls. No association of Val66Met polymorphism with bipolar disorder itself, but with suicidal behavior in bipolar disorder. Mick et al.2009: Family-based association study of 173 bipolar offspring triads. They could not find association of the Val66 allele in children.

3.6.2 NRG1

Neuregulin 1, which is encoded on 8p12, has been identified as a susceptibility factor in schizophrenia and bipolar disorder [Green et al. 2005; Georgieva et al. 2008]. Neuregulin1 is involved in neuronal migration and gliogenesis during brain development. The binding of Neuregulin1 to its receptor erbB is also important for oligodendrocyte development. A loss of NRG1-erbB signaling leads to reduced myelin thickness and slower conduction velocity in CNS axons [Roy et al. 2007]. NRG1 was recently identified as potential candidate in several large genome wide association studies [Segurado et al. 2003; Le-Niculescu et al. 2009; Sklar et al. 2008]. A large family based association study including 515 bipolar participants found association between several SNPs of Nrg1 and bipolar disorder, especially with psychotic manic-depressive-disease [Goes et al. 2009]. Other studies prove evidence of association as well [Green et al. 2005; Perlis et al. 2008]. Green and colleagues prove evidence in a study comprising 529 bipolar and 573 schizophrenic participants in addition to 1011 controls. In contrast, there were also negative results regarding bipolar disorder and this gene [Voineskos et al. 2009]. Nevertheless, there is good evidence for association between NRG1 and bipolar disorder as well as schizophrenia.

3.6.3 NCAM1

NCAM1 (Neural cell adhesion molecule 1) is encoded on locus 11q23.1 and is involved in neuronal growth and maybe in the pathogenesis of bipolar disorder [Arai et al. 2004; Atz et al. 2007]. Already in the 1990s increased levels of neural adhesion molecules were found in the CSF of patients with bipolar disorder [Poltorak et al. 1996].

3.6.4 RELN

The gene RELN codes for a protein, which is important for neurodevelopment. In patients with schizophrenia and bipolar disorder reelin is decreased. Epigenetic changes seem to down regulate reelin gene expression. Hypermethylation in the promoter region of RELN leads to reduced binding of transcription factors and therefore silencing of the gene [Goes et al. 2008].

3.7 Genes of the Lithium signal transduction pathways

3.7.1 DGKH

Diacylglycerol kinase eta (DGKH), a key protein in the lithium-sensitive phosphatidyl inositol pathway, is encoded on 13q14.11. A genome wide association study by Baum and colleagues, including 461 unrelated German bipolar I probands and 562 matched controls as well as a replication study with 772 German bipolar I patients and 876 controls and initial DNA pooling to reduce the costs, showed significant association of DGKH with bipolar disorder (rs1012053, $p = 1.5 \times 10-8$, OR=1.59 in combined samples). The SNP rs1012053 was still significant at the experiment-wide $p<0.01$ after Bonferroni correction of the combined results for the total number of SNPs studied [Baum et al. 2008]. Furthermore, two other genome wide studies showed association between DGKH and bipolar disorder. Since this gene product is involved in lithium sensitive pathways it is not surprising that it shows genome wide association with bipolar disorder [Yosifova et al. 2011; Ollila et al. 2009].

3.8 Ion channels and associated proteins

3.8.1 ANK3

Genes coding for voltage gated ion channels are hot spots for bipolar disorder research, because they were recently identified with high significance in many genome wide association studies [Askland et al. 2009]. Ferreira and colleagues for example found in a 4387 bipolar cases and 6209 controls comprising whole genome scan, a region of very strong association with bipolar disorder which included ANK3 (rs10994336, $P = 9.1 \times 10-9$). ANK3 codes for Ankyrin G, an adaptor protein, which regulates the assembly of voltage-gated sodium channels at axon initial segments [Ferreira et al. 2008]. Additionaly, a meta-analysis of genome scans found significant linkage to chromosomal region 10q11.21-22.1, which overlaps with the location of the ANK3 gene on 10q21. Also a smaller GWAS, which included 1001 European bipolar cases and 1,033 controls, as well as 345 African American bipolar cases and 670 healthy controls supported the role of ANK3 in bipolar disorder [Smith et al. 2009]. Recently, also a meta-analysis of a combined sample of approximately 14 000 subjects of European and Asian-ancestry, as well as a further test in approximately 17 700 cases and controls replicated this association with bipolar disorder [Chen et al. 2011]. Because of replicated association of

ANK3 with manic depressive disease, involvement in pathogenesis of bipolar disorder is highly probable [Segurado et al. 2003; Baum et al. 2008; Ferreira et al. 2008; Scott et al. 2009; Schulze et al. 2009; Smith et al. 2009; Lee et al. 2011, Takata et al. 2011; Gella et al. 2011; Chen et al. 2011; Dedman et al. 2012].

3.8.2 CACNA1C

CACNA1C (located on 12p13.3) codes for the alpha1C subunit of a L-type voltage-gated calcium channel and belongs to the top hits of several GWAS. Recently it has been replicated by diverse GWAS, thus it is undeniable that SNPs of CACNA1C (e.g. rs1006737) play a major role in genetics of bipolar disorder. CACNA1C variants showed strong association with bipolar affective disorder in a whole genome scan by Sklar, which included 1461 bipolar participants and 2008 controls, as well as in a whole genome scan by Ferreira including 4387 cases and 6209 controls (combined P = 7.0 x 10(-8) for CACNA1C SNP rs1006737) [Sklar et al. 2008; Ferreira et al. 2008]. Also pathway-based analysis (PBAs) of Whole genome scans revealed the importance of channelopathies in bipolar disorder [Askland et al. 2009]. CACNA1C variants also seem to be involved in genetics of schizophrenia, major depression and schizotypal personality disorder [Casamassima et al. 2010; Green et al. 2009; Moskvina et al. 2009; Nyegaard et al. 2010; Roussos et al. 2012]. CACNA1C SNPs (e.g. rs1006737) also influence verbal fluency, as well as the memory [Erk et al. 2010; Krug et al. 2010; Zhang et al. 2012; Arts et al. 2013]. Furthermore, some variants of CACNA1C have been associated with structural changes of the CNS for instance significantly increased gray matter volume and reduced functional connectivity within the corticolimbic frontotemporal neural system [Wang et al. 2011]. Recently CACNA1C was again replicated as genome wide significant association in the large-scale-genome-wide-association-analysis of the PGC (Psychiatric GWAS Consortium) in 2011. They conducted a combined GWAS comprising of 7,481 patients with bipolar disorder and 9,250 controls. The replication study tested 34 SNPs in 4,496 independent cases with bipolar disorder and 42,422 independent controls found that 18 of 34 SNPs showed $P < 0.05$, with 31 of 34 SNPs having signals with the same direction of effect ($P = 3.8 \times 10(-7)$). An analysis of all 11,974 bipolar disorder cases and 51,792 controls confirmed genome-wide significant evidence of association for CACNA1C. Additionally, a new intronic variant in ODZ4 was identified [PGC GWAS 2011]. Recently the association between CACNA1C and bipolar disorder was again replicated by Green and colleagues in a new UK sample of 1218 cases with bipolar disorder and 2913 controls which has not been used in any studies previously reported independently or in meta-analyses [Green et al. 2012].

3.8.3 NTNG1 and NTNG2

NTNG1 and NTNG2 are vertebrate specific axon guidance molecules and their expression is reduced in bipolar disorder and schizophrenia. NTNG plays a role in synaptic formation and maintenance [Eastwood et al. 2008].

3.8.4 KCNC2

KCNC2 encodes the Shaw-related voltage-gated potassium channel [The Wellcome trust consortium 2007].

3.8.5 P2RX7/4

P2RX7 is mapped to 12q24.31 and codes for a purinergic ATP-binding calcium channel receptor, which is expressed in the brain. It is involved in 2-arachidonoylglycerol production by microglial cells. It also influences several cells, for example osteoclasts and macrophages [Kapoor et al. 2009]. Significant association exists between the promising Gln460Arg polymorphism of the P2RX7 gene (rs2230912, P2RX7-E13A) and bipolar disorder. This SNP, which leads to a change of the amino acid glutamine to arginine at position 460, is also associated with unipolar disorder [Lucae et al. 2006; Barden et al. 2006; McQuillin et al. 2009; Hejjas et al. 2009]. Other groups tried to replicate this finding recently, but did not succeed [Green et al. 2009; Grigoroiu-Serbanescu et al. 2009]. Further, the microsatellite marker NBG6 was related to bipolar disorder [Shink et al. 2005; Barden et al. 2006; McQuillin et al. 2009]. This gene is a promising candidate since its coding region on chromosome 12q24, lying closeby the chromosomal region of Darier's disease (an autosomal dominant skin disease which cosegregates with affective disorders) has been implicated in several linkage studies of bipolar disorder [Dawson et al. 1995; Ewald et al.1998; Morissette et al.1999; Degn et al. 2001; Maziade et al. 2001; Ewald et al. 2002; Ekholm et al.2003; Green et al. 2005; Shink et al. 2005; Cassidy et al. 2007] and unipolar mood disorder [Abkevich et al., 2003; Zubenko et al. 2003; McGuffin et al. 2005; Lucae et al. 2006].

3.8.6 ATP2A2

ATP2A2, a gene encoding SERCA2-a sarcoplasmic/endoplasmic reticulum calcium pump that plays a role in intracellular calcium signaling, is coded in the susceptibility region for Darier's disease 12q23-q24.1 [Craddock et al. 1993]. Darier's disease is an autosomal dominant skin disease (keratosis follicularis) that cosegregates with affective disorders. This made this region a hot spot for bipolar disorder research. However, some groups showed no evidence for the involvement of ATP2A2 in producing susceptibility to bipolar disorder [Jacobsen et al. 2001; Ruiz-Perez 1999].

3.8.7 SLC24A3

SLC24A3 codes for a potassium dependant sodium/calcium exchanger that plays a critical role in neuronal calcium homeostasis. It was identified in large genome wide linkage study for bipolar disorder with comorbid migraine [Oedegaard et al. 2009].

3.8.8 SLC39A3

SLC39A3 (ZIP3) codes for a channel which is responsible for zinc reuptake. This gene was associated with bipolar disorder in large genome wide association studies [Baum et al. 2009; Olila et al. 2009].

3.9 HPA axis, cortisol and stress

Chronic distress can lead to mood disorders and burnout. Nevertheless, some people can cope better with the same amount of stress than others. Bipolar patients have disturbed cortisol release after stressful events [Watson et al. 2004]. Depressive reaction to stress may be due to special genetic constitution. Certain genotypes lead to enhanced stress response. The ss genotype (patients carrying a pair of short alleles) of the 5-HTTLPR polymorphism in the serotonin transporter promoter region leads for example to enhanced stress reactivity. A very recent study tested this 5-HTTLPR variant in relation to stress response in newborns.

They tested the connection between genotype and cortisol release (a measurement for stress) after a foot prick, which is an element in a routine check, but still associated it with stress for the newborn. SS genotype carriers had much higher cortisol levels than other genotypes. Thus s allele carriers show much higher stress response of the hypothalamus-pituitary-adrenal axis (HPA) than l allele carriers [Müller et al. 2009]. Since chronic stress and stressful events often influence pathogenesis of bipolar disorder, genes involved in the hypothalamic-pituitary-adrenal axis (HPA) are possible susceptibility genes for manic-depressive disease. The HPA is strongly associated with stress response and modulation. The hypothalamus releases CHR binds to CRH receptors in the anterior pituitary gland. In consequence adrenocorticotrophic hormone (ACTH) is released which leads to release of cortisol from the adrenal cortex [Gillespie et al. 2009]. This can be followed by anxiety-related behavior and influences arousal, attention, executive functions, emotions, learning and memory consolidation related to these emotions. So the CRHR1 gene (corticotropin-releasing hormone receptor 1 gene), encoded on 17q12-q22, might be candidate gene for bipolar disorder, although it is not extensively investigated yet. CRHR1 is a G protein-coupled receptor localized in frontal cortical areas, forebrain, brainstem, amygdala, cerebellum, and the anterior pituitary [Refojo et al. 2009]. CRH encoded on 8q13 could be another candidate gene, but the rare genetic studies did not show any evidence [Alda et al. 2000]. Albeit linkage studies showed negative results as well [Stratakis et al. 1997], some genome wide linkage and association studies showed association between the area of 8q13 and bipolar disorder [Liu et al. 2003; Marcheco-Teruel et al. 2006]. Although those genes in HPA might be candidate genes for bipolar disorder, no evidence of association is possible because of great lack of performed studies. However, it might be possible that the HPA system genes are influenced by other susceptibility genes, but are not the underlying cause of pathogenesis. Still, the HPA system and stress response is for sure disturbed in bipolar disorder [Watson et al. 2004].

3.10 Genes of the dopaminergic system

The dopamine system has recently received increased attention in bipolar disorder research. Dopamine was suggested to be involved in pathogenesis of bipolar disorder, because dopamine agonists and precursor can induce mania in high dose. Dopamine antagonists on the other hand have antimanic effects and are used for treatment in manic episodes. Those promanic effects of high-dosed dopamine precursors can be seen in treated patients with Parkinson's disease. There have been case reports of Parkinson patients with switching mood as well. This may implicate a role of dopamine in manic-depressive disease. Dopaminergic hyperactivity is suggested to produce mania, while hypoactivity of the dopaminergic system may lead to depression [Murphy et al. 1971; Cannas et al. 2002]. Dopamine transmits diverse functions including motivation, pleasure, cognition, memory, learning and fine motor control as well as modulation of neuroendocrine signaling. Additionally, dopaminergic transmission is also involved in common mechanism of drugs that leads to addiction [Girault et al. 2004].

3.10.1 DAT1

DAT1 (SLC6A3) encodes for the dopamine transporter, which reuptakes dopamine and, to a minor degree, noradrenaline from the synaptic gap. DAT1 is inhibited by dopamine reuptake inhibitors. The dopamine transporter is encoded on 5p15, which was linked to bipolar disorder by linkage studies [Waldman et al. 1997]. Recently numerous new SNPs in the DAT1 gene and many SNPs and haplotypes have been associated with bipolar disorder [Grünhage et al. 2000]. One of the well-studied -67A/T DAT1 SNP was examined in 136 Iranian bipolar patients and 163 controls. The T allele was associated with bipolar disorder [Keikhaee et al. 2005; Ohadi et al. 2007]. Still, many studies denied an association between DAT1 polymorphisms and bipolar disorder [Souery et al. 1996; Bocchetta et al. 1999]. Another 40bp VNTR in the 3'UTR of DAT1 was also investigated by some studies, however, with negative results [Souery et al. 1996; Bocchetta et al. 1999; Kirov et al. 1999; Heiden et al. 2000; Georgieva et al. 2002]. Recently bipolar disorder with features of ADHD was investigated in 87 families and replicated in 52 bipolar cases and 46 healthy controls. DAT1 may predispose to early prodromal features that include attentional deficits, mood instability and impulsive behavior [Greenwood et al. 2012].

Table 10: Dopamine transporter gene (DAT1) and bipolar disorder

DAT1 polymorphism	Association with BD	No association with BD
40-bp nucleotide repeat polymorphism (VNTR), located in 3'UTR (3' untranslated region)		– Souery et al. 1996 69 bipolar patients and 69 controls from Belgium. – Bocchetta et al. 1999 Family-based association study from Sardinia with 53 bipolar probands and parents. – Kirov et al. 1999 British family association study with 122 bipolar offspring trios. – Heiden et al. 2000 102 Austrian bipolar patients and 79 healthy controls. – Georgieva et al. 2002 Family based association study from Bulgaria with schizophrenia (178 trios), BD (77 trios) and schizoaffective disorder (29 trios).
– 67A/T polymorphism	– Keikhaee et al. 2005 136 Iranian BD patients and 163 controls – Ohadi et al. 2007 240 Iranian BD cases and 213 controls. Association of T-allele with male bipolar patients, but not with females	

3.10.2 DRD1

Dopamine receptors belong to the superfamily of the G-protein-coupled-receptors and can be divided into two major parts; the D1 like receptors comprising of D1 and D5 and the D2 like receptor comprising of D2, D3 and D4 receptors [Emilien et al. 1999]. DRD1 codes for the dopamine 1 receptor and maps to the region 5q35.1. Linkage studies about this region and bipolar affective disorder showed controversial results. While some showed positive results [Garner et al. 2001; Ni et al. 2002; Shink et al. 2002; Sklar et al. 2004], others rejected any linkage [De Bruyn et al. 1994]. A study comprising of 315 bipolar patients, 40 of them with comorbid alcoholism, and 350 controls investigated the relation between the dopamine receptor genes (DRD1-4) and bipolar disorder with and without comorbid alcoholism. Neither, bipolar disorder alone nor bipolar disorder with comorbid alcoholism, were associated with DRD genes [Szczepankiewicz et al. 2007]. A Canadian and Sardinian haplotype analysis showed only trends of association [Del Zompo et al. 2007]. A -48 A/G polymorphism of DRD1, which leads to an A to G exchange at position -48, was associated with bipolar disorder in Sardinian, as well as Polish population [Severino et al. 2005; Dmitrzak-Weglarz et al. 2006]. The -48 A/G polymorphism is also associated with outcome of prophylactic lithium treatment. The G/G genotype leads to poorer response [Rybakowski et al. 2009].

Table 11: DRD1 gene polymorphisms and their relation with bipolar disorder (BD)

Gene polymorphism	Association with BD	No association with BD
– 48 A/G polymorphism	– Severino et al. 2005 107 BD patients and 129 healthy control subjects of exclusively Sardinian descent. – Dmitrzak-Weglarz et al. 2006 407 patients with schizophrenia; 380 patients BD and 399 healthy controls.	– Del Zompo et al. 2007 Sardinian sample: 170 patients with BD and 129 controls. Canadian sample: 229 trios – Szczepankiewicz et al. 2007 317 Polish patients with BD (42 patients with comorbid alcohol abuse) and 350 controls.
– 800T/C polymorphism		– Del Zompo et al. 2007 Sardinian sample: 170 bipolar patients and 129 controls. Canadian sample: 229 trios
1403T/C polymorphism		– Del Zompo et al. 2007 Sardinian sample: 170 patients with BD and 129 controls. Canadian sample: 229 trios

3.10.3 DRD2

DRD2, the dopamine D2 receptor gene, maps to 11q23, a region identified in some linkage studies for schizophrenia and bipolar disorder [Craddock et al. 1999; Serretti et al.1b 2000; Gurling et al. 2001]. Significant positive association between bipolar disorder and allele 5 of the microsatellite polymorphism DRD2 was detected in a large multi-center study [Massat et al. 2002]. Also smaller studies detected association with (CA)n repeat in first intron of DRD2 [Pérez de Castro et al. 1995]. A Chinese study (118 bipolar Han Chinese and 196 controls and, for replication, 157 English and 143 controls) found significant association with the promoter variant and the taq1A polymorphism of DRD2 in Chinese population; yet not in English population [Li et al. 1999]. Further negative results were also shown by other studies [Sasaki et al. 1996; Souery et al. 1996;

Bocchetta et al. 1999; Kirov et al. 1999; Leszczyńska-Rodziewicz et al. 2005; Szczepankiewicz et al. 2007]. The insertion/deletion variant (-141C Ins/Del) in the 5' regulatory region of the dopamine D2 receptor gene is not associated in Caucasians [Stöber et al.1998]. The Ser311Cys polymorphism of DRD2 was significantly associated with mood incongruent psychotic disorder in Japanese and with the symptoms of delusion and disorganization in Italians [Arinami et al. 1996; Serretti et al. 2000]. However, this Ser311Cys SNP was not associated in Japanese and Caucasian studies [Manki et al. 1996; Sasaki et al. 1996; Heiden et al. 2000].

Table 12: DRD2 gene variants and association with bipolar disorder (BD)

DRD2 Polymorphism	Association with BD	No association with BD
TaqA1 polymorphism	– Li et al. 1999: Case-control analysis in 118 bipolar Han Chinese and 196 controls.	– Li et al. 1999: Case-control replication study with 157 bipolar English cases and 143 controls.
Promoter variant	– Li et al. 1999: Case-control analysis in 118 bipolar Han Chinese and 196 controls.	– Li et al. 1999: Case-control replication study with 157 bipolar English cases and 143 controls.
Microsatellite polymorphism (allele 5)	– Massat et al. 2002 Multi-center study of 358 bipolar cases and 358 controls.	– Souery et al. 1996 Sample of 69 bipolar patients and 69 matched controls.
(CA)n repeat in first intron	– Perez de Castro et al. 1995 51 Spanish BD cases and 46 controls.	
-141C Ins/Del polymorphism		– Stöber et al. 1998: A total of 620 unrelated German individuals (260schizophrenics, 70bipolars and 290controls) – Kirov et al. 1999 British family association study with 122 bipolar offspring trios. – Leszczyńska-Rodziewicz et al. 2005 339 Polish BD patients (143 males, 196 females) and 366 controls. – Szczepankiewicz et al. 2007: 317 Polish BD patients (42 patients with comorbid alcohol abuse) and 350 controls.

DRD2 Polymorphism	Association with BD	No association with BD
Ser311Cys polymorphism	– Arinami et al.1996: Japanese case-control study in 291 patients with schizophrenia, 78 patients with affective disorders, and 579 controls. – Serretti et a. 2000: 1182 inpatients (480 BD, 269 major depressive disorder, 366 schizophrenias, 44 delusional disorder, 23 psychotic disorder not otherwise specified) and 267 healthy controls.	– Manki et al. 1996 101 Japanese patients (52 bipolar and 49 unipolar patients) and 100 controls. – Sasaki et al.1996 273 Caucasian patients with schizophrenia, 621 with delusional disorder, 63 BD and 255 controls. – Heiden et al. 2000 102 Austrian BD patients and 79 healthy controls.
TG dinucleotide polymorphism in first intron		– Bocchetta et al. 1999 Family-based association study from Sardinia with 53 bipolar probands and parents.

3.10.4 DRD3

The D3 receptor is of special interest, because it is especially expressed in the limbic area. It is encoded on 3q13.3, an area suggested to be linked to schizophrenia and bipolar disorder [Serretti et al. 2000; Maziade et al. 2001]. BalI RFLP, a DRD3 polymorphism leading to a serine-to-glycine substitution in the first exon, is not associated with bipolar disorder. This claims at least an analysis of 454 bipolar patients and a meta-analysis of previous association studies by Elvidge and colleagues [Elvidge et al. 2001]. Also other association studies pointed out that the DRD3 Ser9Gly polymorphism is not associated with psychosis and bipolar disorder [Shaikh et al. 1993; Manki et al. 1996; Souery et al. 1996; Piccardi et al. 1997; Kirov et al. 1999; Heiden et al. 2000; Elvidge et al. 2001; Leszczyńska-Rodziewicz et al. 2005; Szczepankiewicz et al. 2007; Krelling et al. 2008].

Table 13: DRD3 and bipolar disorder (BD)

Association studies of the DRD3 Ser9Gly polymorphism: NO association with bipolar disorder	
– **Shaikh et al. 1993** 75 BD patients and 79 healthy controls. – **Manki et al. 1996** 101 Japanese patients (52 bipolar and 49 unipolar) and 100 controls. – **Souery et al. 1996** 69 bipolar patients and 69 controls – **Piccardi et al. 1997** Family based study of 44 bipolar probands from Sardinia with both parents. – **Kirov et al. 1999** British family association study with 122 bipolar offspring trios. – **Heiden et al. 2000** 102 Austrian bipolar patients	– **Elvidge et al. 2001** Large English bipolar case control sample (454 BD patients) showed negative results. Additional meta-analysis of 980 bipolar patients and 1100 controls showed no evidence of association between the Ser9Gly polymorphism of DRD3 and bipolar disorder either! – **Leszczyńska-Rodziewicz et al. 2005** 339 Polish BD patients (143 males, 196 females) and 366 controls. – **Szczepankiewicz et al. 2007:** 317 Polish BD patients (42 patients with comorbid alcohol abuse) and 350 controls. – **Krelling et al. 2008** 105 Brazilian women (58 schizophrenic patients and 47 bipolar patients) and 62 gender-matched controls. No association with functional psychosis.

3.10.5 DRD4

DRD4 is located on 11p15.5 and is a highly polymorphic gene. It contains a functional variable number tandem repeat (VNTR) polymorphism in the third exon which consists of 2–10 imperfect tandem repeats of 48 bp and each repeat encoding for 16 amino acids [Van Tol et al. 1992]. The different length polymorphisms reflect different response to clozapine [Van Tol et al. 1991]. This VNTR polymorphism of DRD4 was significantly associated with bipolar disorder [Manki et al. 1996; Muglia et al. 2002], while many other studies could not show this association [Perez de Castro et al. 1994; Oruc 1b et al. 1997; Bocchetta et al. 1999; Li et al. 1999; 1c Serretti et al. 1999; Serretti et al. 2002; Serretti et al. 2004]. Also a SNP, which leads to a C to T exchange at position 521, might not be associated, at least in Polish population [Leszczyńska-Rodziewicz et al. 2005; Szczepankiewicz et al. 2007]. DRD4 was also investigated for delusional symptoms in major psychosis in 2011 inpatients with positive results. The DRD4 exon 3 VNTR polymorphism was significantly associated with delusions [Serretti et al. 1b 1998; Serretti et al. 1d 1999; Serretti et al. 2001]. Also a Mexican association investigation showed evidence of association between the exon 3 and exon 1 polymorphism of DRD4 and psychosis [Aguirre et al. 2007]. The long allele of the exon 3 polymorphism was also associated with certain personality traits including low harm avoidance [Serretti et al. 2006]. Altogether, this is a promising candidate gene for mood disorders, because a meta-analysis (917 patients with bipolar and unipolar patients and 1164 controls) showed significant association between the 48-base-pair- repeat polymorphism and mood disorders in general. Remarkable is that the association between bipolar disorder and the DRD4.2 allele dropped to insignificance after correction for multiple testing. Nevertheless, association between unipolar depression, as well as the combined group (unipolar and bipolar patients together) stayed significant even after Bonferroni correction [Lopez et al. 2005].

Table 14: DRD4 polymorphisms and their association with bipolar disorder (BD)

DRD4 Polymorphism	Association with BD	No association with BD
48-bp-repeat polymorphism in the third exon of DRD4 (VNTR polymorphism)	– Manki et al. 1996 101 Japanese patients (52 bipolar and 49 unipolar) and 100 controls. – Serretti et al. 1d 1999 461 Italian inpatients affected by major psychoses (criteria: mania, depression, delusion and disorganization) were genotyped for DRD4 variants. Exon3 long alleles associated with high delusional score – Serretti et al. 2001 A total of 2011 Italian inpatients! (811 patients with BD, 635 with depression, 419 with schizophrenia, 104 with delusion and 42 psychosis not otherwise specified and 601healthy controls). Long allele is associated with delusion! – Muglia et al. 2002 145 Canadian nuclear families (BD patients and their biological parents). – Lopez et al. 2005 Meta-analysis comprising of 917 patients with unipolar or bipolar disorder and 1164 controls from 12 samples. Significant association even after cor-	– Perez de Castro et al. 1994 64 Spanish patients with BD (25 males and 39 females) and 46controls. – Oruc et al. 1997 83 Croatian BD and unipolar patients bipolars and 71 healthy controls. – Bocchetta et al. 1999 Family-based association study from Sardinia with 53 BD probands and parents. – Li et al. 1999 118 Han Chinese BD patients and 196 controls, replication analysis in 157 English BD cases and 143 controls. – Serretti et al. 1c 1999 Total of 651 Italian inpatients (229schizophrenics, 86 delusionals, 210 bipolars and 126 unipolars and 471 controls). Association between exon3 variants and BD, but not significant after multiple testing correction. – Serretti et al. 2002 Italian family-based association study of 134 nuclear families (103 BD patients and 58 patients with major depressive disorder).

DRD4 Polymorphism	Association with BD	No association with BD
	rection for multiple testing between mood disorders (unipolar and bipolar disorder) and DRD4.2 allele, as well as major depression alone. – Aguirre et al. 2007 149 unrelated Mexican subjects with different kinds of psychosis and 169 healthy cases.	
12 bp-VNTR (exon 1)		– Serretti et al. 1c 1999 Total of 651 Italian inpatients (229 patients with schizophrenia, 86delusion, 210 BD and 126 unipolar depression and 471 controls) – Aguirre et al. 2007 149 unrelated Mexican subjects with different kinds of psychosis and 169 healthy controls
-C521T SNP		– Leszczyńska-Rodziewicz et al. 2005: 339 Polish patients with BD (143 males, 196 females) and 366 controls. – Szczepankiewicz et al. 2007: 317 Polish patients with BD (42 patients with comorbid alcohol abuse) and 350 controls.

3.10.6 DRD5

DRD5 is encoded on 4p16.1, a region implicated in bipolar disorder by early linkage studies [Asherson et al. 1998; Ewald et al. 1998]. Microsatellite markers close to DRD5 show association with schizophrenia, but not with manic-depressive disorder [Muir et al. 2001]. Concording with this, an association by Kirov and colleagues did not find evidence for association. Further studies are necessary since investigation of this gene has been rare [Kirov et al. 1999].

3.11 Genes of the noradrenergic system

3.11.1 NET (SLC6A2)

NET encodes for the noradrenaline transporter, which reuptakes synaptically released noradrenaline as well as dopamine. Noradrenaline transmits diverse effects of the sympathetic nerve system. Noradrenergic transmission is also involved in controlling mood, arousal, memory, learning and pain perception [Kapfhammer et al. 2008]. NET was investigated for its relationship with psychiatric disorders but the results were inconsistent. The silent mutation 1287 A/G in exon 9 of NET is neither associated with bipolar disorder nor with schizophrenia [Leszczyńska-Rodziewicz et al. 2002]. Stöber and colleagues identified 5 missense substitutions; Val69Ile, Thr99Ile, Val245Ile, Val449Ile and Gly478Ser. Yet their association in case control studies for bipolar disorder was lacking [Stöber et al. 1996]. Only F528C might be associated with depressive disorder. As mentioned before NET mediates rapid re-uptake of released noradrenaline into noradrenergic neurons and is one of the main targets of antidepressants which involve NA reuptake inhibition, for instance reboxetine. The F528C polymorphism leads to increased transporter expression and enhanced NA reuptake [Haenisch et al. 2009].

3.12 Genes of the GABAergic system

Gamma-Aminobutyric acid (GABA) is one of the most important inhibitory neurotransmitters in the CNS. GABAergic receptors consist of two main types GABA-A, a ligand-gated inhibitory chloride channel, and GABA-B receptors. GABA-A receptors have 5 subunits and mediate fast synaptic inhibition in the human brain. GABA binds to the beta subunit, while benzodiazepines bind to the alpha subunit, which enhances GABA binding. Some genes have been suggested in genome wide approaches, but studies are lacking. The following is a review about the rare results.

3.12.1 GABRBI

GABRBI, which codes for a subunit of a ligand gated ion channel, namely the GABA-A-receptor, is encoded on 4p12. The polymorphism rs7680321 was associated with bipolar disorder in the GWAS of the Wellcome Trust Consortium

2007. This may implicate a role of the GABA system in mood disorders [Wellcome Trust Consortium 2007].

3.12.2 GABRB2

GABRB2, on 5q34, codes for the beta2-subunit of the gamma-aminobutyric-acid type A receptor. Linkage studies show inconsistent results [Crowe et al. 1999; Ambrosio et al. 2005]. Also alternative splicing at exon -10 and the resulting different isoforms influence risk for psychotic disorders [Zhao et al. 2009].

3.12.3 GABRB3

GABRB3 is coded on Xq28, which was suggested to be linked with bipolar disorder in many genome wide approaches and smaller linkage studies [Baron et al. 1994; Wigg et al. 2009]. A European multicenter study with 185 bipolar participants and 370 controls showed association between the dinucleotide polymorphism and female bipolar patients [Massat et al. 1b 2002]. The CA repeat polymorphism was not associated with bipolar disorder in a small Greek sample [Papadimitriou et al. 2001].

3.12.4 GABRA5

GABRB5 on 15q11-q13 codes for the alpha5 subunit of the GABA-A receptor and might influence pathogenesis of bipolar disorder. Polymorphism IVS1-21G>A and some haplotypes are associated with manic-depressive disease, at least in Japanese population [Otani et al. 2005]. The 282-bp allele of a dinucleotide (CA) repeat was significantly associated with dominance of manic episodes [Papadimitriou et al. 1998].

3.13 Genes of the Glutamatergic system

3.13.1 GRIN genes

GRIN1, on chromosome 9q34.3, codes for the zeta-1 subunit of NMDA receptors. Mundo and colleagues showed association between GRIN1 and bipolar disorder in a family association study comprisinging 288 patients with their parents [Mundo et al. 2003]. GRIN2B is located on 12p12 and was associated in some linkage and association studies for bipolar disorder [Fallin et al. 2005; Martucci et al. 2006; Avramopoulos et al. 2007; Lorenzi et al. 2009; Lorenzi et al. 2010]. Nevertheless, a very recent study consisting of 419 bipolar patients and 487 controls could not show association [Szczepankiewicz et al. 2009]. GRIN2C is encoded on 17q25 and GRIN2D on 19q13.1-qter was only associated in one family-based association study comprising of 101 trios and 203 quads from bipolar Caucasian families. Through lack of further studies association has to be handled with caution [Shi et al. 2008].

3.13.2 GRIA1

GRIA1 located on 5q31.1 codes for the ionotropic glutamate receptor AMPA1, which has been associated with cognitive functions, for example memories. This locus was significantly linked to bipolar disorder in a Latin-American linkage study [Herzberg et al. 2006]. GRIA1 was as well associated with manic-depressive disorder in Shi's family based on an association study [Shi et al. 2008]. Also, GRIA1 was recently associated with psychotic bipolar disorder [Kerner et al. 2009].

3.13.3 GRM3

GRM3, a metabotropic glutamate receptor gene located on 7q21.1-q21.2, was associated with bipolar disorder in a Jewish study by Fallin. Meanwhile, Marti and colleagues could not find any association with it in a German sample [Marti et al. 2002; Fallin et al. 2005]. Albeit one genome wide linkage approach also showed linkage to 7q21, replication studies are absolutely necessary since studies are lacking [Minnis et al. 2003].

3.13.4 GRM4

GRM4, on 6p21.3, codes for the metabotropic glutamate receptor 7. Fallin and colleagues found association between GRM4 and bipolar disorder but further association studies are lacking [Fallin et al. 2005].

3.13.5 GRM7

Glutamate neurotransmission was implicated to play a major role in bipolar disorder as it belonged to the top hits of the Wellcome Trust Consortium GWAS in the year 2007. Polymorphism rs1485171 in the GRM7 (metabotropic glutamate receptor 7) gene, encoded on 3p26.1-p25.1, showed significant association (P=9.7×10-5) with this disease in the joint GWAS which included 2,000 British individuals for each of 7 major diseases (bipolar disorder, coronary artery disease, Crohn's disease, hypertension, rheumatoid arthritis, type 1 diabetes and type 2 diabetes) and a shared set of 3,000 British controls [Wellcome Trust Consortium 2007].

3.13.6 GRIK genes

GRIK4, on 11q22.3, codes for the glutamate receptor KA1 that was associated with bipolar disorder recently [Pickard et al. 2008]. The glutamate receptor KA2 is coded on the GRIK5 gene on 19q13.2 and was associated with bipolar disorder in a large study about substance abuse, anxiety, eating, psychotic and mood disorders and comprised 3214 samples. Also a small GWAS comprising of 88 bipolar disorder patients and 376 control subjects showed nominal association in the combined sample of GWAS and replication study [Gratacos et al. 2009; Yosifova et al. 2011].

3.14 Copy number variations (CNVs)

Structural variations in DNA from one kilobase (kb) to several megabases (Mb), which are called copy number variations, are responsible for the bigger part of interindividual heterogeneity of the genome and are still underestimated. CNVs are quantitative variations in the genome including tandem arrays of repeats, as well as submicroscopic deletions and duplications. They are created by retrotransposition, which duplicates and inserts some coding and non-coding DNA segments randomly around the genome. Some CNVs interrupt genes and can thus disturb their functions, but the bigger part does not affect physiology at all [Redon et al. 2006; Lachman et al. 2008; Conrad et al. 2009]. Single nucleotide polymorphisms often reside next to copy number variations and may be a hint for finding new SNPs responsible for bipolar disorder. Even top candidates of large genome wide association studies (DGKH, SORCS2, DFNB31, A2BP1, and

NXN) are affected by polymorphic copy number variations [Baum et al. 2008; Lachman et al. 2008]. DGKH, DFNB31, A2BP1, and NXN influence the Wnt/GSK3I3 signaling pathway, a lithium inhibited pathway. GSK3β itself is affected by several copy gain and copy loss variants [Lachman et al. 2007]. A complex CNV at 15q13–14 containing a polymorphic inversion involving CHRNA7 and its fusion variant CHRFAM7A was also associated with bipolar disorder [Flomen et al. 2008]. Another study by Wilson detected copy number variations in genes involved in glutamate signaling [Wilson et al. 2006]. A recent study by Zhang and colleagues who examined singleton CNVs in bipolar disorder, copy number variations occurring once in a dataset, made following gene discoveries: GRM7, DLG2, SOX5, LARGE [Zhang et al. 2009]. There are also many diseases based on deletions, insertions or transversions in genes or chromosomal areas (CNVs), which cosegretate with bipolar disorder. Those disorders can be a possibility to find new susceptibility genes for mood disorders. The 3-megabase microdeletion on 22q11 in VCFS (velocardio facial syndrome), a congenital disorder associated with heart disease, cleft palate and very often schizophrenic or bipolar symptoms, helped to identify the COMT gene predisposing for mood disorder and schizophrenia [Craddock et al. 2009]. A 1:11(q42.1; q14.3) translocation, which disrupts the DISC1 gene, is another major cytogenetic mutation that influences bipolar disorder as well as schizophrenia [Murphy et al. 1999; Millar et al. 2000; Blackwood et al. 2001; Kas et al. 2009].

3.15 Others

3.15.1 GCHI

GCHI codes for a GTP-cyclohydrolase, which is the rate-limiting enzyme in the biosynthesis of tetrahydrobiopterin, a natural cofactor for tyrosine and tryptophan hydroxylases. GCHI is located on 14q22-24; a region that was identified as bipolar disorder susceptibility locus in whole genome scans of linkage and meta-analysis of genome scans as well as association and linkage studies [Segurado et al. 2003; Kaeley et al. 2005; Liu et al. 2003; Cassidy et al. 2007; Zhao et al. 2007].

3.15.2 CHMP1.5

CHMP1.5 on 18p11.2 encodes for a chromatin modifying protein and lies within a chromosomal region, which has been linked to bipolar disorder in whole genome scans and linkage studies performed in patients with bipolar disorder. McNabb and colleagues could not find any association between two SNPs (rs1786581 and rs1249624) in 402 bipolar individuals and 181 unrelated controls, only a slight trend towards association. They suggested that the region 18p11.2, linked to bipolar disorder, might include another susceptibility gene instead of CHMP1,5 [Detera-Wadleigh et al. 1999; McNabb et al. 2005; Segurado et al. 2003].

4. Genetic overlaps between psychiatric diseases

Since Kraepelin divided affective disorders and schizophrenia in two distinct categories nobody has ever questioned the Kraepelinian dichotomy, although both diseases share at least psychosis. Nowadays, however, genetic discoveries argue that bipolar affective disorder and schizophrenia are more related than assumed before. To determine whether boundaries between schizophrenia and bipolar disorder are blurred one must elucidate the genes, which are shared by both diseases [Lin et al. 2008].

4.1 Overlaps between mood disorders and schizophrenia

4.1.1 Schizophrenia

Already over 150 years ago Kraepelin described schizophrenia as "dementia praecox "[Peters et al. 2006]. Then Eugen Bleuler (1857-1939) coined the term schizophrenia. Kurt Schneider, a German psychiatrist and a pupil of Karl Jaspers, divided the symptoms into first and second rank. First rank symptoms comprised of audible thoughts, arguing voices, commenting voices, experience of influences playing on the body, thought withdrawal, thought insertion, thought diffusion (also called thought broadcast) and delusional perception. Modern classifications include fundamental symptoms of Bleuler and Schneider. Since some decades the symptomatology distinguishes between positive and negative symptoms. Positive symptoms are delusions and hallucinations, while negative ones are flattening of affect, poor planning, more generally expressed, lowering of energetic potential [Tölle 2008]. The etiology and pathophysiology of schizophrenia is not exactly known, but it is for sure multifactorial. A combination of neurobiochemical, neuroanatomic and genetic alterations lead to disease. The classical "dopamine hypothesis" states that schizophrenia is based on "dopaminergic hyperactivity". But there are also imbalances in the serotonin-, glutamate- and

GABA-systems [Kapfhammer et al. 2008]. Beside biological factors, one should not forget psychosocial and environmental factors. These factors lead to disease outbreak, if there is an underlying genetic susceptibility for schizophrenia. Schizophrenia has a very strong genetic predisposition. Heritability is as high as 80% [Norton et al. 2006; Burmeister 2008]. The genetic endowments of schizophrenia are proven by many twin, adoption and family studies. The concordance rate for monozygotic twins lies around 50%, while it is only 10% for fraternal twins, whereas the average person has only a risk of 0,5-1,6% to fall ill with schizophrenia [Rothenhäusler 2007]. Among the various already discovered genes that lead to schizophrenia, there are still numerous unkown ones. The following genes showed nominal evidence of association with schizophrenia in a meta-analysis recently: APOE, COMT, DAO, DRD1, DRD2, DRD4, DTNBP1, GABRB2, GRIN2B, HP, IL1B, MTHFR, PLXNA2, SLC6A4, TP53 and TPH1 [Allen et al. 2008]. DRD2 (11q23.1), GABRB2 (5q34), DTNBP1 (6p22.3), IL1B (2q13) and COMT (22q11.21) were proven to be associated in a meta-analysis of genome scans of schizophrenia either [Lewis et al. 2003].

4.2 Overlaps between mood disorders and schizophrenia

4.2.1 Symptomatic overlaps between psychiatric diseases

The most overlapping feature between schizophrenia and bipolar affective disorder is psychosis. Over 50% of patients classified with bipolar affective disorder experience at least one psychotic episode during their lifetime [Coryell et al. 2001]. Affective symptoms are another overlap. Schizophrenic patients have affective symptoms similar to those in mood disorders. Negative symptoms, for example anhedonia, are similar to depressive ones. Schizophrenic patients may exhibit reduced emotional responses or experience hyperactive and exultant feelings like manic patients. There are also overlaps in medication. Atypical antipsychotics that target the dopamine 2 (D2) and serotonin 5-HT2A-receptors can be used in patients with schizophrenia, as well as bipolar patients. Since those drugs are effective in both disorders this implicates that the dopaminergic and serotonergic pathways may be involved in the pathogenesis of both disorders [McIntyre et al. 2007; Rothenhäusler 2007; Bishara et al. 2009; McFadden et al. 2009; Tohen et al. 2009; Fountoulakis et al. 2010]. Bipolar and unipolar disorder share symptoms too. Depressive symptoms can occur in major depression, as well as in bipolar disorder during depressive states. Another common feature is suicidality. Patients with mood disorders or schizophrenia experience suicidal ideation at some point of the disease or even try to commit suicide. So there is a great possibility that those diseases are genetically related [Rothenhäusler 2007].

4.2.2 Genetic overlaps between mood disorders and schizophrenia

Schizophrenia research has reached many achievements recently. The schizophrenia GWAS consortium investigated 21,856 European patients with schizophrenia in the first stage and 29,839 independent subjects with schizophrenia in the second replication stage in the year 2011. The schizophrenia GWAS consortium found seven loci (1p21.3, 2q32.3, 8p23.2, 8q21.3, 10q24.32-q24.33, 6p21.32-p22.1 and 18q21.2) with genome wide significance. MIR137 (rs1625579) was the strongest new finding ($P = 1.6 \times 10^{-11}$) and codes for a regulator of neuronal development. Beside CACNA1C (rs4765905, $P = 7.0 \times 10^{-9}$), ANK3 (rs10994359, $P = 2.5 \times 10^{-8}$) and the ITIH3-ITIH4 region (rs2239547, $P = 7.8 \times 10^{-9}$) reached genome wide significance in a joint analysis with a bipolar disorder sample (16,374 patients with bipolar disorder or schizophrenia and 14,044 controls) either [Schizophrenia Psychiatric GWAS Consortium 2011]. Furthermore hundreds of association and linkage studies have been conducted. Some overlaps between mood disorders and schizophrenia are discussed in this chapter.

COMT

The COMT gene is located at 22q11, which lies in the deleted region of the congenital velocardiofacial syndrome (VCFS). This syndrome includes cleft palate, heart disease, cognitive and learning impairments, as well as high risk for schizophrenia and bipolar disorder. The VCFS microdeletion increases the risk for schizophrenia by the 30 to 50-fold! The highest known risk factor for schizophrenia, beside having either parents or a monozygotic twin with the disease, is the deletion of VCFS at 22q11 [Murphy et al. 1999]. Patients with velocardiofacial syndrome show a schizophrenia rate around 24%, which made the gene in this region to a top target for schizophrenia research [Hamilton et al. 2008]. Many association studies supported the relationship between COMT gene variants and schizophrenia, especially the Val158Met polymorphism [Lewis et al. 2003; Shifman et al. 2004; Fan et al. 2005; Funke et al. 2005; Allen et al. 2008; Chien et al. 2009; Brisch et al. 2009; Wang et al. 2009; Hoenicka et al. 2020]. Even a large meta-analysis comprising 2628 schizophrenic participants and 7340 controls prove association between COMT gene variants and schizophrenia [Allen et al. 2008]. Despite the successful results, there have been also negative outcomes as for instance in a recent Japanese meta-analysis, which denied association [Okochi et al. 2009]. COMT is not only a promising susceptibility gene for schizophrenia, but also for bipolar disorder. Goghari and colleagues showed that the well-investigated Val158Met polymorphism is associated with psychotic symptoms in bipolar disorder and schizophrenia [Goghari et al. 2008]. Also further association studies prove evidence of COMT involvement in bipolar affective disorder [Lachman et al. 1996; Kirov et al. 1998; Shifman et al. 2004; Funke et al. 2005; Burdick et al. 2007; Goghari 2008; Zhang et al. 2009]. Altogether COMT is a very important risk gene for schizophrenia and bipolar disorder [Kunugi et al. 1997; Frisch et al. 1999; Baekken et al. 2008; Waray et al. 2008]. Yet, Massat and colleagues found that the Val/Val genotype of the Val158Met polymorphism is associated with early onset depressive disorder [Massat et al. 2005].

Serotonin transporter polymorphisms

SERT (=5HTT = serotonin transporter gene)

The gene coding for the serotonin transporter (5-HTT) has been a hot spot of mood disorder research for several decades, since this transporter is the main target of the effective and widely used SSRI. Decrease of synaptic serotonin during depressive episodes is a central element of the monoamine hypothesis of depression. Therefore the serotonin transporter, which reuptakes serotonin from the synaptic gap, is the most attractive candidate gene. Efficiency of 5-HTT-mediated inward and outward transport is enhanced in depressed patients [Willeit et al.2008].

VNTR in intron 2 of the serotonin transporter gene

Already 14 years ago this variable number tandem repeat polymorphism was the center of interest in renowned scientific magazines including the Lancet. The 9 repeat allele of this 5-HTTVNTR was associated with major affective disorder by Ogilvie and colleagues [Ogilvie et al. 1996], which was confuted in the same year by a Japanese group [Kunugi et al. 1996]. Haplotype analyses recognized certain haplotypes that comprise a special VNTR in intron2 and a deletion in the promoter region to be associated with depression [Gutierrez et al. 1998]. Nevertheless, there are results, which negate any association of this VNTR in intron 2 and depression in Chinese people [Yen et al. 2003]. Results in bipolar disorder research are also conflicting. Many association studies claim involvement of the intron 2 VNTR polymorphism in manic-depressive disease [Collier et al. 1996; Craddock et al. 1996; Battersby et al. 1996; Kunugi et al. 1996; Rees et al. 1997;

Bellivier et al. 1998; Furlong et al. 1998; Kirov et al. 1999; Bellevier et al. 2002]. Almost the same amount showed negative results in bipolar disorder [Stöber et al. 1996; Hoehe et al. 1998; Bocchetta et al. 1999; Vincent et al. 1999; Olivieira et al. 2000; Saleem et al. 2000; Mellerup et al. 2001; Dimitrova et al. 2002; Yen et al. 2003; Alaerts et al. 2009]. Also schizophrenia has a good chance to be associated with this polymorphism. A meta-analysis, comprising of 12 population-based-association-studies consisting of 2177 cases and 2369 control subjects, showed that the 12-repeat allele was significantly associated with schizophrenia [Fan et al. 2005]. Also another meta-analysis for schizophrenia showed association with this polymorphism. Conflicting results may be due to small study sizes and different ethnic populations [Allen et al. 2008].

Deletion/insertion in the promoter region of SERT

A 44 base pair insertion/deletion polymorphism in the 5' regulatory region of the serotonin transporter gene (5-HTTLPR) has been center of research for decades. Association between the polymorphism and depression was observed in many studies. A large German study, comprising of 466 patients and 836 controls, prove that the short allele of the 5-HTTPLR polymorphism is significantly associated with major depressive disorder. The short allele, containing the deletion, leads to reduced transcriptional activity of the promoter, which consequently reduces the rate of expression by 30–40% [Heils et al. 1995; Hoefgen et al. 2005]. Also subtypes of depression were investigated. Melancholic depression was associated with the 5-HTTLPR s-allele and atypical depression with the l allele [Willeit et al. 2003]. In addition seasonal affective disorder was also associated with the s-allele [Rosenthal et al. 1998; Sher et al. 1999]. Altogether there are many studies, which favor an association between depression and the s-allele or haplotypes [Gutierrez et al. 1998; Hauser et al. 2000]. However, among a large meta-analysis there are also other studies denying any association [Frisch et al. 1999; Serretti et al. 1999; Lasky-Su et al. 2005]. Besides, there is a possibility that the short allele is associated with suicidal behavior, which can be part of many diseases [Neves et al. 2008]. Schizophrenia was also investigated for this polymorphism, but the 5-HTTLPR insertion/deletion polymorphism is not likely to be involved in pathogenesis. This claims at least a large meta-analysis [Fan et al. 2005]. Results in bipolar depression are again controversial. The majority of the studies shows no evidence of association [Kunugi et al. 1996; Collier et al. 1996; Rees et al. 1997; Esterling et al. 1998; Hoehe et al. 1998; Mendes de Oliviera et al. 1998; Geller et al. 1999; Kirov et al. 1999; Serretti et al. 1999, Vincent et al. 1999; Olivieira et al. 2000; Ospina-Duque et al. 2000; Bellivier et al. 2002; Serretti et al. 2002; Mendlewicz et al. 2004; Neves et al. 2008; Vincze et al. 2008; Alaerts et al. 2009; Mick et al. 2009]. Nevertheless next to two meta-analysises are other studies that show a possible factor in pathogenesis of bipolar disorder [Bellivier et al. 1998; Rotondo et al. 2002; Anguelova et al. 2003; Hauser et al. 2003; Lasky-Su et al. 2005; Meira-Lima et al. 2005].

G72/G30 gene (DAOA)

DAOA is located at 13q13-q14 and codes for the D-amino acid oxidase activator. Many studies suggest evidence of association with bipolar disorder [Bass et al. 2009; Fallin et al. 2005; Schulze et al. 2005; Maziade et al. 2009], however, some do not [Shi et al. 2008; Gomez et al. 2009; Maheshwari et al. 2009]. Furthermore, this gene may confer risk to schizophrenia [Zou et al. 2005; Allen et al. 2008; Bass et al. 2009; Maziade et al. 2009; Shi et al. 2008; Shi et al. 2009]. A large Japanese multicenter study with 1774 patients with schizophrenia and 2092 healthy controls found association with several SNPs that did not survive correction for multiple testing [Ohi et al. 2009]. Moreover, other association studies neglected relation to schizophrenia [Jönsson et al. 2009]. DAOA may also confer risk to major depressive disorder, but studies are lacking. Nevertheless, G72 was associated with major depression and neuroticism [Rietschel et al. 2008].

DAO

DAO might confer susceptibility to schizophrenia, bipolar disorder and unipolar disorder [Fallin et al. 2005; McGuffin et al. 2005; Schulze et al. 2005; Allen et al. 2008; Rietschel et al. 2008; Shi et al. 2008; Wirgenes et al. 2009]. Yet some association studies neglected association of DAO with schizophrenia and bipolar disorder [Bass et al. 2009; Jönsson et al. 2009].

CACNA1C

CACNA1C codes for the alpha1C subunit of the L-type voltage-gated calcium channel. This top susceptibility gene is significantly associated with bipolar disorder. This was proven by several large genome wide association studies and their meta-analysis [Ferreira et al. 2008; Sklar et al. 2008; Moskvina et al. 2009; Askland et al. 2009]. CACNA1C also seems to be associated with major depression and schizophrenia [Green et al. 2009; Moskvina et al. 2009; Casamassima et al. 2010; Green et al. 2010; Nyegaard et al. 2010; Schizophrenia GWAS Consortium 2011].

DTNBP1

DTNBP1 on chromosome 6p22.3 is coding for the protein dysbindin or dystrobrevin binding protein1 and is one of the most important susceptibility genes for schizophrenia [Lewis et al. 2003; Breen et al. 2006; Duan et al. 2007; Allen et al. 2008; Réthelyi et al. 2009; Wessman et al. 2009; Wirgenes et al. 2009]. Dysbindin is part of the dystrophin complex and has functions in synaptic plasticity and signal transduction. This complex regulates for example nicotinic receptor clustering and recruits specific signaling molecules such as neuronal nitric oxide synthase and also interacts with postsynaptic density proteins involved in *N*-methyl-D-aspartate (NMDA) receptor clustering. Defects in this gene product could lead to problems in synaptic transmission and postsynaptic receptor regulation [Miyamoto et al. 2003]. Only a small number of studies for schizophrenia showed negative results for this gene [Jönsson et al. 2009]. This susceptibility gene might be another overlap with bipolar disorder [Fallin et al. 2005; Breen et al. 2006; Pae et al. 2007; Gaysina et al. 2009]. Nevertheless, it is not likely to play a role in major depressive disorder [Zill et al. 2004].

Neuregulin1

Neuregulin1, which is encoded on 18p12, is strongly associated with susceptibility for schizophrenia [Green et al. 2005; Lachman et al. 2006; Georgieva et al. 2008; Réthelyi et al. 2009]. However, there are association studies with negative results [Jönsson et al. 2009]. Manic-depressive disease shares this susceptibility gene with schizophrenia [Segurado et al. 2003; Green et al. 2005; Georgieva et al. 2008; Perlis et al. 2008; Sklar et al. 2008; Goes et al. 2009; Le-Niculescu 2009]. Major depressive disorder was also not associated in a large-scale study with almost 1400 depressed participants and 1300 controls [Schosser et al. 2010]. Neuregulin1 functions in neuronal migration and brain development. It is associated with several neurotransmitter systems for instance the NMDA-, glutamate- and GABA-system [Miyamoto et al. 2003].

DISC 1

DISC-1 and DISC-2 (Disrupted in schizophrenia 1 and 2) are risk genes for schizophrenia. Both genes are disrupted by a balanced 1:11 translocation and they reside at 1q42.1 [Miyamoto et al. 2003]. The mutation leads to altered neuronal structure and cognition [Kvajo et al. 2008]. DISC1 is involved in cytoskeletal, synaptogenic and neurodevelopmental functions [Duan et al. 1b 2007; Hennah et al. 2009]. The translocation leads to a truncated DISC protein, which leads to a deletion at the carboxy-terminal end. The DISC1 protein seems to play a role in cortical development. This may happen through interactions with NUDEL and LIS1 proteins, which are important in neuronal migration [Kamiya et al. 2006]. DISC1 regulates proliferation and differentiation of neuronal progenitor cells via

GSK3beta/beta-catenin signaling. A suppression of DISC1 leads to reduced neuronal proliferation [Mao et al. 2009]. The DISC1 locus was identified in a genome wide linkage scan for schizoaffective disorder, as well as bipolar disorder [Macgregor et al. 2004; Hamshere et al. 2006]. Among numerous studies a recent meta-analysis supported evidence of association between schizophrenia and DISC1 [Hodgkinson et al. 2004; Saetre et al. 2008; Schumacher et al. 2009; Tomppo et al. 2009]. Nevertheless, many studies doubt this association [1b Kim et al. 2008]. Thus DISC1 might be another overlap between both diseases [Hodgkinson et al. 2004; Macgregor et al. 2004; Maeda et al. 2006; Palo et al. 2007; Le-Niculescu 2009; Schosser et al. 2010].

BDNF

BDNF is a promising and well studied candidate gene for bipolar disorder [Sklar et al. 2002; Neves-Pereira et al. 2002; Geller et al. 2004; Lohoff et al. 2005; Green et al. 2006; Vincze et al. 2008; Xu et al. 2009; Liu et al. 2008; DeLuca et al.2008; Fan and Sklar 2008; Le-Niculescu 2009]. It might be associated with schizophrenia and major depressive disorder either [Watanabe et al. 2007; Schumacher et al. 2005]. A meta-analysis showed evidence of association between the BDNF C270T polymorphism and schizophrenia [Watanabe et al. 2007]. On the other hand a Japanese meta-analysis recently rejected association of the two most important BDNF variants with schizophrenia [Kawashima et al. 2009], as well as a meta-analysis for major depression denied association with BDNF [Chen et al. 2008].

MAOA

MAOA gene variants seem to be associated at some degree with all three psychiatric diseases. Yu and colleagues showed significantly increased frequency of the 4-repeat allele of the promoter VNTR polymorphism of MAOA in major depressed patients [Yu et al. 2005]. The more active longer allele of the MAO-A VNTR was significantly associated with complicated grief in the female subgroup of patients [Kersting et al. 2007]. Some association studies supposed a connection of MAO variants and schizophrenia [Jönsson et al. 2003; Qiu et al. 2009]. However, a meta-analysis stated that there is no association between the variable number tandem repeat (VNTR) polymorphism and the T941G polymorphism and schizophrenia [Norton et al. 2002; Li et al. 2008]. Syagailo and colleagues showed no association between the MAOA-LPR variant and susceptibility to recurrent major depression, bipolar disorder and schizophrenia in our population [Syagailo et al. 2001]. The CA repeat microsatellite polymorphism of intron2 and the -941T->G SNP are suggested to be associated with bipolar disorder [Furlong et al. 1999; Kawada et al. 1995; Rubinsztein et al. 1996; Lim et al. 1995; Preisig et al. 2000], although those two polymorphism had also negative study results [Parsian and Todd 1997; Preisig et al.2000; Lin et al. 2008; Serretti et al. 2002; Craddock et al. 1995; Muramatsu et al.1997; Nöthen et al. 1995].

Dopamine receptor genes

DRD1

Recently DRD1 was associated with schizophrenia in a meta-analysis [Allen et al. 2008], but there are also association studies that show negative results in schizophrenic patients [Kojima et al. 1999]. DRD1 has also a conflicting role in bipolar disorder, as well as in unipolar disorder. Although some association studies show positive results for bipolar disorder [Severino et al. 2005; Dmitrzak-Weglarz 2006], others presented negative results. Since studies are lacking, further studies are necessary to find the role of DRD1 in mood disorders, [Savoye et al. 1998; Del Zompo 2007; Szczepankiewicz 2007].

DRD2

DRD2 might be a susceptibility gene for schizophrenia and bipolar disorder, although results are inconsistent. There are some positive results for bipolar disorder [Perez de Castro et al.1995; Arinami et al.1996; Li et al. 1999; Serretti et al. 2000; Massat et al. 2002; Serretti et al. 2000], but there are also many results, which lead to a doubt of association with manic depressive disease [Souery et al. 1996; Stöber et al. 1998; Manki et al. 1996; Sasaki et al. 1996; Furlong et al. 1998; Savoye et al. 1998; Bocchetta et al. 1999; Kirov et al. 1999; Li et al. 1999; Heiden et al. 2000; Leszczyńska-Rodziewicz et al. 2005; Szczepankiewicz et al. 2007]. DRD2 seems not to play a major role in major depressive disorder [Furlong et al. 1998]. While some meta-analysis showed evidence of association for the DRD2 gene with schizophrenia, evidence for mood disorder is inconsistent, [Gurling et al. 2001; Lewis et al. 2003; Allen et al. 2008; Serretti et al. 2000].

DRD3

There is overwhelming evidence that DRD3 polymorphisms are not important for development of bipolar disorder [Savoye et al. 1998; Shaikh et al. 1993; Manki et al. 1996; Souery et al. 1996; Piccardi et al. 1997; Kirov et al. 1999; Heiden et al. 2000; Elvidge et al. 2001; Rodziewicz et al. 2005; Szczepankiewicz et al. 2007; Krelling et al. 2008]. Additionally, the rare studies for unipolar disorder show negative results [Manki et al. 1996]. Existing studies suggest association of DRD3 with schizophrenia [Talkowski et al. 2006; Dominguez et al. 2007], however, the bigger part of the studies neglected a relation. Concording with these large case control studies, not even Japanese and Chinese meta-analysises could find a relation between schizophrenia and D3 dopamine receptor gene variants, especially the Ser9Gly polymorphism [Lorenzo et al. 2007; Fathalli et al. 2008; Ma et al. 2008; Utsunomiya et al. 2008; Nunokawa et al. 2010]. So maybe all three diseases have in common, that they are not associated with DRD3.

DRD4

DRD4 seems to play a major role in schizophrenia and bipolar disorder, but not in major depression [Oruc et al. 1997; Firsch et al. 1999]. There are much more supporting studies for bipolar disorder than unipolar disorder [Manki et al. 1996; Serretti 1b et al. 1998; Serretti 1d et al. 1999; Serretti et al. 2001; Muglia et al. 2002; Lopez et al. 2005; Aguirre et al. 2007] and there are even more negative results in association studies for bipolar disorder [Perez de Castro et al. 1994; Oruc et al. 1b 1997; Bocchetta et al. 1999; Li et al. 1999; 1c Serretti et al. 1999; Serretti et al. 2002; Serretti et al. 2004; Leszczyńska-Rodziewicz et al. 2005]. Recently Schizophrenia was associated with DRD4 variants in a meta-analysis [Allen et al. 2008], but again, there are also negative results for schizophrenia and bipolar disorder [Oruc et al. 1997].

DRD5

Schizophrenia and manic-depressive disorder show evidence of association with the dopamine receptor D5 gene. Further studies are lacking [Asherson et al. 1998; Ewald et al. 1998; Muir et al. 2001; Pal et al. 2009].

4.3 Summary of the overlaps between mental diseases

Table 16: Excerpt of overlapping candidate genes of schizophrenia and mood disorders (BD and MD)

	Association with schizophrenia	Association with bipolar disorder (BD)	Association with unipolar depression (MD)
COMT	Lewis et al. 2003 (meta-analysis) Shifman et al. 2004 Fan et al. 2005 (meta-analysis) Funke et al. 2005 Abdolmaleky et al. 2006 Allen et al. 2008 (meta-analysis) Chien et al. 2009 Brisch et al. 2009 Hoenicka et al. 2010 (in Spanish males) Wang et al. 2009 Bhakta et al. 2012	Lachman et al.1996 Kirov et al. 1998 Shifman et al. 2004 Funke et al. 2005 Abdolmaleky et al. 2006 Burdick et al. 2007 Goghari et al. 2008 Abdolmaleky etl. 2009 (epigenetic study) Zhang et al. 2009 (large association study and meta-analysis on 19studies) Lee et al. 2010 Benedetti et al. 2011 Nohesara et al. 2011 (Epigenetic study) Lelli-Chiesa et al. 2011 (BD and emotional pro-gressing)	Ohara et al. 1998 Massat et al. 2005 Schosser et al. 2012 (suicidality in treatment resistant major depres-sion) Aberg et al. 2010 (in Swedish men with MD) Comasco et al. 2011 (postpartum depression) Massat et al. 2011
MAOA	Jönsson et al. 2003 Qiu et al. 2009 (only in men)	Furlong et al. 1999 (meta-analysis) Kawada et al. 1995 Rubinsztein et al. 1996 Lim et al. 1995 Preisig et al. 2000 Fan et al. 2010 (meta-analysis)	Yu et al. 2005 Zhang et al. 2009 Fan et al. 2010 (meta-analysis) Comasco et al. 2011 (postpartum depression) Lung et al. 2011 (suicide attempts in depressed male)
DISC1	Hodgkinson et al. 2004 Hamsgire et al. 2005 Saetre et al. 2008 Schumacher et al. 2009 (association study and meta-analysis) Tomppo et al. 2009 Ram Murthy et al. 2012 (sex dependant)	Rubinsztein et al. 1996 Furlong et al. 1999 Blackwood et al. 2001 Thomson et al. 2005 Hamshere et al. 2005 Maeda et al. 2006 Müller et al. 2007 Palo et al. 2007 Müller et al. 2007 Hennah et al. 2009 Le-Niculescu et al.2009 Schosser et al. 2010 Xiao et al. 2011	Hashimoto et al. 2006 Schosser et al. 2010 Thomson et al. 2012

	Association with schizophrenia	Association with bipolar disorder (BD)	Association with unipolar depression (MD)
		(in Chinese) Ram Murthy et al. 2012 (sex dependant)	
DRD1	Allen et al. 2008 (meta-analysis) Lee et al. 2011 Zhu et al. 2011	Severino et al. 2005 Dmitrzak-Weglarz et al. 2006	Cannon et al. 2009
DRD2	Serretti et al. 2000 Gurling et al. 2001 Lewis et al. 2003 (meta-analysis) Allen et al. 2008 (meta-analysis) Cordeiro et al. 2009 Fan et al. 2010 Sáiz et al. 2010 Liu et al. 2012 (Japanese) Voisey et al. 2012 Zheng et al. 2012	Perez de Castro et al.1995 Arinami et al. 1996 Li et al. 1999 Serretti 2000 Massat 2002 Serretti et al. 2000	Wang et al. 2012
DRD4	Allen et al. 2008 (meta-analysis) Shi et al. 2008	Manki 1996 Serretti 1b 1998 Serretti 1d 1999 Serretti 2001 Muglia 2002 Lopez 2005 Aguirre 2007	Manki et al. 1996 Xiang et al. 2008
DRD5	Muir et al. 2001 Pal et al. 2009	Asherson 1998 Ewald et al. 1998	Lack of studies
GABRB2	Lewis et al. 2003 (meta-analysis) Allen et al. 2008 (meta-analysis) Shi et al. 2008	Crowe 1999	Lack of studies
GRIN2B	Allen et al. 2008 (meta-analysis)	Fallin et al. 2005 Avramopoulos Szczepankiewicz et al. 2009	Lack of studies
NRG1	Green et al. 2005 Lachman et al. 2006 Georgieva et al. 2008 Réthelyi et al. 2009 Yang et al. 2012 Agim et al. 2013 (analysis of 3GWAS)	Segurado et al. 2003 Green et al. 2005 Walss-Bass et al. 2006 Georgieva et al. 2008 Perlis et al. 2008 Sklar et al. 2008 Goes et al. 2009 Le-Niculescu 2009 Prata et al. 2009	Lack of studies

	Association with schizophrenia	Association with bipolar disorder (BD)	Association with unipolar depression (MD)
NCAN	Mühleisen et al.2012	Cichon et al. 2011	Lack of studies
MTHFR	Arinami et al. 1997 Kempisty et al. 2007 Allen et al. 2008 (meta-analysis) Shi et al. 2008	Kempisty et al. 2007	Arinami et al. 1997 McGuffin et al. 2005
CACNA1C	Green et al. 2009 Moskvina et al. 2009 Nyegaard et al. 2010 Hamshere et al. 2012 (GWAS) Schizophrenia Psychiatric GWAS Consortium 2011 (GWAS)	Ferreira et al. 2008 (GWAS, P=7.0 x 10(8)) Sklar et al.2008 (GWAS) Askland et al. 2009 (GWAS) Sklar et al. 2011 (GWAS, genome wide-significance) PGC GWAS 2011 (GWAS, genome-wide significance) Green et al. 2012 (GWAS) Arts et al. 2013 (cognitive functioning in BD) Radua et al. 2012 (emotional processing and BD)	Green et al. 2009 Casamassima et al. 2010
ANK3	Athanasiu et al. 2010 Schizophrenia Psychiatric GWAS Consortium 2011 (GWAS) Yuan et al. 2012	Segurado et al. 2003 (meta-analysis of genome scans) Baum et al. 2008 (GWAS) Ferreira et al. 2008 (GWAS, P=9.1 x 10(-9)) Scott et al. 2009 (meta-analysis of GWAS) Schulze et al. 2009 Smith et al. 2009 (GWAS) Lee et al. 2011 (GWAS) Takata et al. 2011 Gella et al. 2011 Chen et al. 2011 (meta-analysis of GWAS) Dedman et al. 2012	Lack of studies
APOE	Digney et al. 2005 Allen et al. 2008 (meta-analysis) Dean et al. 2008	Bellivier et al. 1997 Digney et al. 2005 Dean et al. 2008	Lack of studies

	Association with schizophrenia	**Association with bipolar disorder (BD)**	**Association with unipolar depression (MD)**
BDNF	Neves-Pereira et al.2005 Rosa et al. 2006 Watanabe et al. 2007 (meta-analysis)	Sklar et al. 2002 Neves-Pereira et al. 2002 Geller et al. 2004 Lohoff et al. 2005 Green et al. 2006 Liu et al. 2008 DeLuca et al.2008 Sklar et al. 2008 Le-Niculescu et al. 2008 (GWAS analysis) Liu et al. 2008 Vincze et al.2008 Xu et al. 2009 Xu et al. 2010 Sears et al. 2011 Ivanova et al. 2012 Wang et al. 2012	Schumacher et al. 2005 Hilt et al. 2007 Li et al. 2013 (treatment resistant depression)
SERT/5HTT	Chotai et al. 2005 Fan et al. 2005 (meta-analysis) Allen et al. 2008 (meta-analysis) Shi et al. 2008	Bellivier et al. 1998 Rotondo et al. 2002 Anguelova et al. 2003 (meta-analysis) Hauser et al. 2003 Lasky-Su et al. 2005 (meta-analysis) Meira-Lima et al. 2005 Manchia et al. 2010 Neves et al. 2010 (violent suicide attempts in BD) Sugawara et al. 2011 (Epigenetics analysis in concordant monocygotic twins)	Battersby et al. 1996 Ogilvie et al. 1996 Hauser et al. 2000 Willeit et al. 2003 Hoefgen et al. 2005 Dong et al. 2009 Rucci et al. 2009
TPH	Chotai et al. 2005 Zaboli et al. 2006 Allen et al. 2008 (meta-analysis)	Chen et al. 2008 Bellivier et al. 1998	Gizatullin et al. 2006
DTNBP1	Lewis et al. 2003 (meta-analysis) Breen 2006 Duan et al. 2007 Allen et al. 2008 (meta-analysis) Réthelyi et al. 2009 Wessman et al. 2009 Wirgenes et al. 2009	Fallin et al. 2005 Breen 2006 Joo et al. 2007 Pae et al. 2007 Gaysina et al. 2009	Lack of studies

	Association with schizophrenia	**Association with bipolar disorder (BD)**	**Association with unipolar depression (MD)**
DAO	Allen et al. 2008 (meta-analysis) Shi et al. 2008 Wirgenes et al. 2009	Fallin et al. 2005 Schulze et al. 2005	McGuffin et al. 2005 (GWAS)
DAOA	Zou et al. 2005 Allen et al. 2008 (meta-analys) Bass et al. 2009 Maziade et al. 2009 Shi et al. 2008 Shi et al. 2009	Fallin et al. 2005 Schulze et al. 2005 Bass et al. 2009 Maziade et al. 2009	Rietschel et al. 2008

5. Gene-environment-interactions and prevention

5.1 Epigenetics

Lifestyle and environmental factors, including diet, drugs, alcohol and hormones, can influence inherited features without changing DNA sequence, however, with epigenetic changes, including methylation, acetylation, ubiquitination and phosphorylation of DNA or histones. Thus environment has an impact on inheritability and gene regulation with chemical modification of DNA segments (e.g. promoters), which are important for gene expression. Especially cytosine in so-called CpG islands, which are located especially in regulatory elements, gets methylated. The methyl group is provided by S-adenosyl methionine. Hypermethylation of promoters lead to silencing of the gene or reduced transcription, irreversible if very densely methylated [Bogdanovic et al. 2009]. Potentially all genes of our genome could be expressed in every cell, because every cell carries the whole genome inside. However, since cells are specialized and adaption to environment is important, not all genes are necessary and some must be silenced. This happens along with other mechanisms by epigenetic modification. Those chemical changes are performed by many host enzymes. DNA methyltransferases are responsible for DNA methylation, and histones are modified by histone acetyltransferases (HATs), histone deacetylases (HDACs), as well as methyltransferases and demethylases [Abdolmaleky et al. 2004; Connor et al. 2008]. Many neurodevelopmental and neuropsychiatric diseases, including Prader Willi und Angelman syndrome, are influenced by epigenetic changes and genomic imprinting [Horstthemke et al. 2008]. Epigenetic changes, for example pathological increased CpG methylation and repressive chromatin remodeling at 5' regulatory sequences, might also be a cause for heritable susceptibility to bipolar disorder [Connor et al. 2008; Mill et al. 2008]. Methylation of the promoter regions of BDNF, DRD2, REELN, HTR2A and other genes lead to predisposition for bipolar disorder. Also genes of the glutamatergic and GABAergic system with epigenetic modification lead to vulnerability for psychiatric diseases [McGowan et al. 2008; Mill et al. 2008]. Hypomethylation of the COMT promoter, leading to enhanced expression of the enzyme, is responsible for increased predisposition for bipolar disorder and schizophrenia [Abdolmaleky et al. 2006; Connor et al. 2008]. Nevertheless, this is also in doubt [Dempster et al. 2006]. Epigenetic changes of REELN confer susceptibility for bipolar disorder and schizophrenia. Hypermethylation of the REELN promoter leads to decreased expression of Reelin, which is important for neuronal migration and synaptogenesis [Abdolmaleky et al. 2004; Abdolmaleky et al. 2005]. Aberrant methylation status was also identified in twins disconcordant for bipolar disorder. Especially the X-chromosome showed different patterns of methylation [Rosa et al. 2008].

5.2 Sleep deprivation

Sleep deprivation has antidepressant effects and can lead to a switch of mood in bipolar patients. Yet it leads to better brightening of mood in long allele carriers of the SERT promoter deletion/insertion polymorphism [Benedetti et al. 1999].

5.3 Nutrition and famines

Famines lead to reduced protein synthesis and in consequence to oligodendrocyte cell loss and hypomyelination. Many proteins involved in nerve growth are coded by genes and are disturbed in bipolar affective disorder. So hunger might affect especially bipolar patients with certain genetic predisposition [Carter et al. 2007]. Acute tryptophan depletion leads to reduced transient serotonergic neurotransmission and negative mood [Nugent et al. 2008; Robinson et al. 2009]. Special variants of the serotonin transporter gene lead to different response to this depletion of tryptophan. The short allele of 5-HTTLPR, a 44bp insertion/deletion polymorphism in the 5' regulatory region of the serotonin transporter gene (SLC6A4) leads, especially in relationship with tryptophan depletion and positive family history, to depression. While the ss genotype leads more frequently to depression during tryptophan depletion, the ll genotype is protective [Neumeister et al. 2002; Firk et al. 2009]. Totally opposing results show another small study. They suggest the ll genotype to lead to depressive response during tryptophan depletion [Moreno et al. 2002].

5.4 Infections and risk of bipolar disorder

Infections might increase the risk of mood disorders. Already in the late 1970s the Bornavirus, which cause a rare meningoencephalitis, was highly discussed to play a role in mood disorders and many studies showed Bornavirus antibodies and antigenes in patients with affective disorder [Pini et al. 1996; Salvatore et al. 1997; Ferszt et al. 1999; Bode et al. 2001; Terayama et al. 2003]. Amantadine treatment reduces mania in bipolar patients infected with Bornavirus [Ohlmeier et al. 2008]. Also HSV-1 could be considered. HSV-1 infection and COMT Val158Met polymorphism affect cognitive functioning in individuals with bipolar disorder [Dickerson et al. 2006]. Nevertheless nowadays infections are not highly discussed in pathogenesis of bipolar disorder, but chronic inflammatory disease based on oxidative stress and immunological mechanisms are hot spots of research today.

5.5 Season of birth

The season of birth is a well-replicated environmental factor for development of bipolar disorder, maybe because infections occur more often in winter and spring [Torrey et al. 1996; Mino et al. 2000]. Chotai and colleagues investigated the connection between season of birth and gene variants of tryptophan hydroxylase (TPH), serotonin transporter (5-HTTLPR) and dopamine receptor (DRD4) with positive results [Chotai et al. 2003].

5.6 Urban/rural residency and genotype

A study by Jokela claims that urban residency is associated with low depressive symptoms in Finnish individuals carrying the T/T or T/C genotype of the T102C polymorphism of HTR2A, whereas not in those carrying the C/C genotype. The T allele was associated with high depressive symptoms in remote rural areas, but with low depressive symptoms in urban or suburban areas [Jokela et al. 2007].

5.7 Antidepressant induced mania and genotypes

Antidepressants can lead to a switch to manic symptoms, especially with a predisposing genotype. Carriers of the short allele of 5-HTTLPR are prone to get antidepressant-induced mania [Mundo et al. 2001; Ferreira et al. 2009]. Nevertheless, no association was found in a study of 305 bipolar patients between the 44bp insertion/deletion polymorphism in the 5-HTTLPR of the serotonin transporter with antidepressant-induced-mania [Rousseva et al. 2003]. Children and youths with bipolar disorder do not show any association between the serotonin transporter promoter polymorphism and antidepressant induced mania. Yet especially young people, irrespective of genotype, are at risk and should be observed when given antidepressants [Baumer et al. 2007].

5.8 Stress, gene expression and bipolar disorder

Chronic stress or stressful events can lead to mood disorders and burnout, but not everybody is affected by it the same way. People cope differently with distress. While some people put away stress easily, others react exaggeratedly. This may all be due to genetic predisposition and personality traits. Certain genotypes of serotonergic system related genes lead to greater susceptibility for depressive disorder after stress exposure, because they modulate the acute serotonergic reaction to the stressor [Holmes et al. 2009]. The ss genotype of 5-HTTLPR, a regulatory region of the serotonin transporter gene, leads to depressive reaction after stress exposure, while ll allele carriers are protected against depression [Eley et al. 2004; Kendler et al. 2005; Firk et al. 2009]. The ss genotype of the 5-HTTLPR polymorphism also leads to enhanced stress reactivity in general. A very recent study tested the 5-HTTLPR variant in relation to stress response in newborns. They tested the relation between genotype and cortisol release after a foot prick, which is an element in a routine check, but is still associated with stress for the newborn. SS genotype carriers had much higher cortisol levels than other genotypes. Thus s allele carriers show much higher stress response than l allele carriers [Müller et al. 2009]. Stress and glucocorticosteroids lead to decreased expression of BDNF in the brain, especially the hippocampus [Smith et al. 1995]. Not only leads chronic unpredictable stress to reduced serotonergic firing, but it also leads to desensitization of 5-HT1A autoreceptors. Altogether it is proven that chronic stress induces mood instabilities and especially genetically predisposed people should try to reduce stress and find good coping strategies [Bambico et al. 2009].

5.9 Mood changes after delivery

The so called "baby blues" is a widespread depressive episode in the postpartum period, which may be influenced by certain gene variants. Not only depressive episodes can occur, but also psychosis is an issue in postpartum period. Especially women with bipolar disorder are at special risk for psychosis after delivery. Almost half of bipolar women get puerperal psychosis some days after delivery [Coyle et al. 2000]. After childbirth there is a sharp reduction in tryptophan availability in the brain, thus polymorphic variations in 5-HTT may play a role in the post-partum psychosis. High expression 5-HTT genotypes (ll genotype) might be a risk factor under certain environmental conditions such as tryptophan depletion after childbirth [Sanjuan et al. 2008]. Also other groups show that certain 5-HTTLPR polymorphism of the serotonin transporter influence the susceptibility to puerperal psychosis [Coyle et al. 2000]. A genome wide linkage study for postpartum mood disorder identified the regions 1q21.3-q32.1 with KCNN3 and 9p24.3-p22.3 as hot spots. Within the fine-mapping study the gene HMCN1 at 1q25.3-q31.1 reached the best results [Mahon et al. 2009].

5.10 Maltreatment and negative life events

Maltreatment in childhood is a severe trauma, which leads very often to psychological problems in adulthood. Nevertheless, some victims can cope better than others with similar childhood experiences. Therefore there might be some protective genotypes that help to prevent outbreak of depression or other psychiatric disease [Caspi et al. 2002].

5.10.1 MAOA polymorphism

While maltreated children sometimes grow up and develop antisocial behavior and victimize people around them, others do not. Caspi and colleagues found that the functional promoter polymorphism of the MAOA gene moderates the effect of maltreatment. Polymorphisms, which lead to high levels of monoamine oxidase, were protective against antisocial behaviour, while carriers of polymorphisms, which produce low activity MAOA, were likely to invent violent behavior in their adulthood after maltreatment experience in their childhood. So genotypes seem to moderate children's sensitivity to environmental insults [Caspi et al. 2002]. Other groups showed that low activity MAO is associated with anti-social behavior after traumatic life events including not only maltreatment, but also a parent's death, parent's marital problems or other emotional difficult events [Frazzetto et al. 2007].

5.10.2 Hypothalamic-pituitary-adrenal axis

The hypothalamic-pituitary-adrenal-axis (HPA) is strongly associated with stress response and modulation. The hypothalamus releases CHR, which binds to CRH receptors in the anterior pituitary gland. In consequence adrenocorticotrophic hormone (ACTH) is released leading to a release of cortisol from the adrenal cortex [Gillespie et al. 2009]. Specific CRHR1 polymorphisms appear to moderate the effect of child abuse on the risk for adult depressive symptoms [Bradley et al. 2008; Bet et al. 2009; Tyrka et al. 2009]. Polanczyk and colleagues reported that the TAT haplotype, comprising of 3 CRHR1 SNPs, is protective against developing depression after childhood maltreatment [Polanczyk et al. 2009].

5.10.3 FKBP5

FKBP5 polymorphisms are associated significantly with childhood abuse followed by post-traumatic stress disorder in adulthood. Additionally, certain FKBP5 genotypes influence glucocorticoid receptor sensitivity [Binder et al. 2008].

5.10.4 Serotonin transporter 5-HTTLPR polymorphism

The short (s) less active allele of the serotonin transporter 5-HTTLPR polymorphism was associated with a greater risk of adult depression in the presence of a history of either childhood maltreatment or multiple life events in a 5-year period before onset [Brown et al. 2008]. Also a large prospective-longitudinal study published in Science showed the same results. More depressive results occurred in ss genotype carriers after recent life traumas than in carriers with a set of two "long alleles" of the 5HTTLPR polymorphism. Therefore homozygosity of long alleles is protective against depressive reaction after traumatic life events [Caspi et al. 2003]. Also Kendler, as well as Kaufman and colleagues, showed enhanced depressive reaction to life events in ss genotype carriers [Kaufman et al. 2004; Kendler et al. 2005]. A Swedish cohort of 1482 students at the age of 17-18 years was investigated for the relationship between depression, maltreatment and genotype. The association between maltreatment and depression alone was significant in both genders, while the association with the ss genotype was only significantly associated in girls [Aslund et al. 2009]. Totally opposite results reached a study over 247 young adult female twins. The results showed significantly more depressive reactions to life traumata in long allele carriers [Chorbov et al. 2007]. Also a recent Chinese study showed that 5-HTTLPR polymorphisms influence the reaction to negative life events in the same way [Zhang et al. 2009]. So genetic predisposition might be an explanation why stressful experiences lead to major depression in some people, but not in others. Although special genotypes confer high risk to depression after maltreatment, special social support can help ss genotype carriers to reach very low depression scores. Positive social environment can recover negative experiences in childhood, even with ss genotype [Kaufman et al. 2004].

5.10.5 BDNF

Also BDNF variants lead to more depressive reaction after maltreatment or other life events. The met allele of the BDNF Val66Met variant leads especially in combination with two short alleles of the 5-HTTLPR deletion polymorphism to very high depression scores after maltreatment. Nevertheless, social support lowered the risk very much, even in ss genotype carriers [Kaufman et al. 2004; Kaufman et al. 2006].

5.10.6 COMT

COMT polymorphisms were investigated for a relation between high emotionality in children following maternal postpartum depressive symptoms and adverse life events for children in a large English longitudinal study comprising of 8511 children recently. Maternal postpartum depression and traumatic life events increases the risk of high emotionality of children, but this does not correlate with any COMT genotype [Evans et al. 2009].

5.11 Implications for clinical practice

5.11.1 Treatment and genotype

Antidepressant treatment and genotype

Different genotypes of certain gene variants involved in molecular pathogenesis of affective disorders lead to different treatment results. The ss genotype of the serotonin transporter promoter polymorphic region leads to poor response to SSRI [Serretti et al. 2004]. Also other gene variants influence antidepressant efficacy. The A218C TPH polymorphism was associated with slower response to fluvoxamine in the AA carrier [Serretti et al. 2001]. COMT polymorphisms also influence antidepressant response. The Val/Val genotype of the COMT val158met polymorphism leads to worse effects of antidepressant treatment [Baune et al. 2008]. Since genotypes influence efficacy of therapy, genotyping could be a means for planning therapy in the future. This would personalize treatment decisions and would help to give the right effective medication even to non-responders. The results of genetic research may help to construct guidelines for antidepressant or antimanic chronic treatment. Of course this is still far from clinical practice but, might become true in the future [Luddington et al. 2009].

Antimanic treatment and genotype

Response to lithium is associated with certain genotypes of susceptibility genes. Also the -48 A/G polymorphism of the dopamine receptor D1 gene is associated with outcome of prophylactic lithium treatment. The G/G genotype leads to poorer response [Rybakowski et al. 2009]. Serotonin transporter gene polymorphisms, like the s allele of the 5-HTTLPR, influence Lithium treatment outcome as well. Non-responders had significantly more ss genotypes [Rybakowski et al. 2005], while the ls genotype shows better response [Serretti et al. 2004]. BDNF polymorphisms, for instance the Val66Met polymorphisms, are also associated with Lithium response [Rybakowski et al. 2005]. A combination of s-alleles of the 5-HTTLPR and Val/Val genotype of the BDNF Val66Met polymorphism leads for example to non-response during Lithium treatment [Rybakowski et al. 2007].

5.11.2 Psychotherapy

Body and mind are not independent entities. The brain creates our mind and our mind influences our body. Emotions can influence gene expression via hormonal response, signal transduction and epigenetic changes and thus stressful life events can influence mental health. For example fear leads to arousal of the sympathetic nervous system, which leads to enhanced gene expression of ACTH and cortisol, which in consequence influences several reactions of our body. Thus our way of life leads to epigenetic changes which can be inherited because of methylation or acetylation of DNA or histones. Already Engel pleaded in 1977 for the bio-psycho-social paradigma which includes all 3 dimensions of human life; the biological, psychological and sociological interacting aspects [Engel 1978]. Since our way of life, our feelings and emotions can change gene expression of susceptibility genes, psychotherapy might be an important preventive weapon against bipolar disorder, especially with a genetic predisposition. It might be a helpful tool to resolve stress and childhood traumata and may help to influence gene expression and epigenetic changes in a positive way. Therefore not only genes can influence our susceptibility toward depression or mania, but also our way of life and our emotions can influence how often and how fast certain genes are transcribed and expressed [Abdolmaleky et al. 2004; Connor et al. 2008; Bogdanovic et al. 2009].

5.11.3 Lifestyle changes

Lifestyle changes may help to prevent manic or depressive episodes. Extreme sleep deprivation, which can trigger manic episodes especially with genetic predisposition to bipolar disorder, should be avoided if possible. So shift work, excessive going out or staying up extremely late is counterproductive. A well regulated sleep-wake-cycle will help to prevent manic episodes triggered by extreme sleep deprivation and will reset the molecular clock, which is often disturbed in patients with mood disorders. Another way to influence our daily rhythms is light therapy. This might be of additional benefit especially in wintertime. Clock genes expression is also disturbed by obesity [Kaneko et al. 2009]. So loosing weight might help to reorganize the clock gene system. Especially sport would help here, because sport is not only helpful for loosing weight, but also influences BDNF (Brain Derived Neurotrophic Factor) in a positive way, which increases neurogenesis and antidepressant effects [Sylvia et al. 2009]. Healthy nutrition with a balanced protein, carbohydrate and vegetable intake might help to loose weight and to prevent depressive episodes. Tryptophan depletion and glucose depletion leads especially in some allele carriers to depressive reactions. Therefore a well balanced diet might be partly beneficial. Even to eat at regular times would help as a timekeeper for the circadian system [Mendoza et al. 2006]. Chronic stress is another point which should be considered. Extreme dystress over long periods can trigger depressive episodes especially with a predisposing genotype. So everything stress resolving might be useful: autogenic training, sports or better time management.

Table 17: Gene environment interactions leading to mood disorders or aggravation of symptoms and possibility of treatment and prevention

Gene-environment-interaction influencing affective disorders	**Supporting studies**	**Prevention and treatment**
Obesity	Kaneko et al. 2009	Loosing weight: Healthy and balanced diet Sport
Stress	Eley et al. 2004 Kendler et al. 2005 Firk et al. 2009 Holmes et al. 2009 Müller et al. 2009 Bambico et al. 2009	Sport Coping strategies Mental training Psychotherapy Social support Time management
Maltreatment	Caspi et al. 2003 Kendler et al. 2005 Kaufman et al. 2006 Chorbov et al. 2007 Brown et al. 2008 Aslund et al. 2009	Prevention! Careful look on depressed children. Early interaction. Social support and psychotherapy helps to moderate the risk of affective disorders after childhood maltreatment.
Winter/Summer	Christensen et al. 2008 Volpe et al. 2006 Volpe et al. 2008 Volpe et al. 2009	Light therapy SSRI
Season of birth	Torrey et al. 1996 Mino et al. 2000 Chotai et al. 2003	
Urban/ rural residency	Jokela et al. 2007	Moving to more relaxing spot
Smoking	Saiyad et al. 2012	Stopping smoking
Famines and nutrition	Carter et al. 2007	Balanced healthy diet Enough proteins, carbo-hydrates and vitamins
Tryptophan depletion	Neumeister et al. 2002	
Sleep deprivation/ shift work	Meyrer et al. 2009	Sleep hygiene Avoiding excessive going out- Avoiding shiftwork
Delivery	Sanjuan et al. 2008	Professional support after delivery if necessary

6. Conclusion

Bipolar disorder is a highly heritable disease, which has been proven by many family, twin and adoption studies, as well as modern genetic approaches. A long list of possible susceptibility genes has been discovered so far (see page 21). Interestingly top candidates belong to the Ion channel group and Ion channel associated proteins- especially ANK3 and CACNA1C are favorite predisposing genes. CACNA1C codes for the alpha1C subunit of the L-type voltage-gated calcium channel and influences verbal fluency aside from other important functions. ANK3 codes for an adaptor protein, which regulates the assembly of voltage-gated sodium channels at axon initial segments. Until now both genes show genome wide significant evidence of association with bipolar disorder. Another promising chapter of bipolar disorder research is the growth hormone group. BDNF seems to be associated with bipolar disorder in Caucasians, but not in Asians. BDNF could even be a laboratory marker for bipolar disorder because serum levels are decreased in manic, depressed and euthymic states of manic-depressive disease. BDNF is responsible for neuronal development, synapse formation, serotonergic axon growth, memory acquisition and consolidation, and antidepressant effect, therefore a role in pathogenesis of bipolar disorder is not unlikely. A further candidate gene group includes the "clock genes", including ARNTL, CRY1 and 2, PER1-3. Changes in circadian rhythms are typical features in mood disorders. This goes along with the positive study results for many "clock gene" polymorphisms in smaller association studies, but not in recent GWAS. Although everybody would expect the serotonin system to play a major role, the serotonin receptor genes are not very likely to influence bipolar disorder a lot. The very well examined serotonin transporter polymorphisms are more likely to be involved in pathogenesis of manic-depressive disease (even though they did not belong to genome wide associations of large GWAS either). Also other neurotransmitter systems, for example the dopamine and noradrenaline system, do not show overwhelming results. The genes of the GABA and glutamate system have not been highly investigated yet, but show some positive results. Beside those well examined gene groups, a huge list of new detected genes exists. Some might have been found just by chance, so further investigation is necessary to clarify the role of the candidate genes. Nevertheless, the benefits of molecular psychiatry research are beyond question. Many gene variants are related with bad treatment response or depressive reaction after maltreatment in childhood, for example the short allele of the 5-HTTLPR deletion polymorphism. Those detected gene-environment-interactions can help to tailor individual therapy plans in the future. Genetic knowledge also helps to clarify nosology. Boundaries between psychiatric diseases are blurred. Schizophrenia, bipolar and unipolar disorders share a huge amount of susceptibility genes (see chapter 5). Although hundreds of genes have been discussed, one must not be too enthusiastic. We are still far from elucidation of the underlying mechanism of bipolar disorder. Even though bipolar disorder has a strong genetic background and although association studies, as well as linkage studies have been carried out for decades, findings are still inconsistent. It may be due to small study sizes. GWAS including participant numbers as common in Schizophrenia research nowadays are needed to finally elucidate the true susceptibility genes. Up to 10 000 participants have been recently suggested by the PGC (Psychiatric Genetics Consortium). It could be also due to population stratification. There have been totally diverging results in Asian and Caucasian studies. Future studies have to account for different allele frequencies in different populations and even for gender differences. Another reason for conflicting results might be that bipolar disorder by itself could be an inhomogenous disease with several subtypes and maybe different susceptibility genes. Perhaps even every single individual patient has a unique constellation of variations of susceptibility genes and this could lead to converging study results. It may also just not be possible to find evidence for association for exactly one susceptibility gene variant. Maybe a group of gene variants must be investigated for its risk to lead to bipolar disorder. Much more combinations have to be tested.

Isn't it a possibility that we have to say goodbye to strict boundaries of psychiatric disease that existed for centuries? Maybe borders are even more fluent than we think at the moment. As we could see there are strong genetic overlaps between bipolar affective disorder, schizophrenia and unipolar depression. Maybe Kraepelin's dichotomy of psychosis in schizophrenia and bipolar disorder is not valid anymore [Craddock et al. 2005]. Finally we must admit that psychiatric genetics is still in its infancies and we have to overcome teething troubles.

7. References

A:

Abdolmaleky HM, Smith CL, Faraone SV, Shafa R, Stone W, Glatt SJ, Tsuang MT (2004) Methylomics in psychiatry: Modulation of gene-environment interactions may be through DNA methylation.Am J Med Genet B Neuropsychiatr Genet 127B(1):51-9.

Abdolmaleky HM, Cheng KH, Russo A, Smith CL, Faraone SV, Wilcox M, Shafa R, Glatt SJ, Nguyen G, Ponte JF, Thiagalingam S, Tsuang MT (2005) Hypermethylation of the reelin (RELN) promoter in the brain of schizophrenic patients: a preliminary report. Am J Med Genet B Neuropsychiatr Genet 134B(1):60-6.

Abdolmaleky HM, Cheng KH, Faraone SV, Wilcox M, Glatt SJ, Gao F, Smith CL, Shafa R, Aeali B, Carnevale J, Pan H, Papageorgis P, Ponte JF, Sivaraman V, Tsuang MT, Thiagalingam S. Hypomethylation of MB-COMT promoter is a major risk factor for schizophrenia and bipolar disorder. Hum Mol Genet. 2006 Nov 1;15(21):3132-45. Epub 2006 Sep 19.

Abdolmaleky HM, Cheng KH, Faraone SV, Wilcox M, Glatt SJ, Gao F, Smith CL, Shafa R, Aeali B, Carnevale J, Pan H, Papageorgis P, Ponte JF, Sivaraman V, Tsuang MT, Thiagalingam S.Hypomethylation of *MB-COMT* promoter is a major risk factor for schizophrenia and bipolar disorder.Hum Mol Genet. Author manuscript; available in PMC 2009 December 30.

Abdolmaleky HM, Yaqubi S, Papageorgis P, Lambert AW, Ozturk S, Sivaraman V, Thiagalingam S. Epigenetic dysregulation of HTR2A in the brain of patients with schizophrenia and bipolar disorder. Schizophr Res. 2011 Jul;129(2-3):183-90. doi: 10.1016/j.schres.2011.04.007. Epub 2011 May 7.

Åberg E, Fandiño-Losada A, Sjöholm LK, Forsell Y, Lavebratt C.The functional Val158Met polymorphism in catechol-O-methyltransferase (COMT) is associated with depression and motivation in men from a Swedish population-based study. J Affect Disord. 2011 Mar;129(1-3):158-66. doi: 10.1016/j.jad.2010.08.009. Epub 2010 Sep 9.

Abkevich V, Camp NJ, Hensel CH, Neff CD, Russell DL, Hughes DC, Plenk AM, Lowry MR, Richards RL, Carter C, Frech GC, Stone S, Rowe K, Chau CA, Cortado K, Hunt A, Luce K, O'Neil G, Poarch J, Potter J, Poulsen GH,

Saxton H, Bernat-Sestak M, Thompson V, Gutin A, Skolnick MH, Shattuck D, Cannon-Albright L (2003) Predisposition locus for major depression at chromosome 12q22-12q23.2. Am J Hum Genet 73(6):1271-81. Epub 2003 Nov 5.
Abrahamson EE., Moore RY (2001) Suprachiasmatic nucleus in the mouse: retinal innervation, intrinsic organization and efferent projections. Brain Research 916: 172-191
Agim ZS, Esendal M, Briollais L, Uyan O, Meschian M, Martinez LA, Ding Y, Basak AN, Ozcelik H.Discovery, validation and characterization of erbb4 and nrg1 haplotypes using data from three genome-wide association studies of schizophrenia. PLoS One. 2013;8(1):e53042. doi: 10.1371/journal.pone. 0053042. Epub 2013 Jan 3.
Aguirre AJ, Apiquián R, Fresán A, Cruz-Fuentes C (2007) Association analysis of exon III and exon I polymorphisms of the dopamine D4 receptor locus in Mexican psychotic patients. Psychiatry Res 153(3):209-15. Epub 2007 Sep 5.
Alda M, Turecki G, Grof P, Cavazzoni P, Duffy A, Grof E, Ahrens B, Berghöfer A, Müller-Oerlinghausen B, Dvoráková M, Libigerová E, Vojtěchovský M, Zvolský P, Joober R, Nilsson A, Prochazka H, Licht RW, Rasmussen NA, Schou M, Vestergaard P, Holzinger A, Schumann C, Thau K, Rouleau GA (2000) Association and linkage studies of CRH and PENK genes in bipolar disorder: a collaborative IGSLI study. Am J Med Genet 96(2):178-81.
Alaerts M, Venken T, Lenaerts AS, De Zutter S, Norrback KF, Adolfsson R, Del-Favero J (2006) Lack of association of an insertion/deletion polymorphism in the G protein-coupled receptor 50 with bipolar disorder in a Northern Swedish population. Psychiatr Genet 16(6):235-6. Abstracts
Alaerts M, Ceulemans S, Forero D, Moens LN, De Zutter S, Heyrman L, Lenaerts AS, Norrback KF, Goossens D, De Rijk P, Nilsson LG, Adolfsson R, Del-Favero J (2009) Detailed analysis of the serotonin transporter gene (SLC6A4) shows no association with bipolar disorder in the Northern Swedish population. Am J Med Genet B Neuropsychiatr Genet 150B(4):585-92.
Allen NC, Bagade S, McQueen MB, Ioannidis JP, Kavvoura FK, Khoury MJ, Tanzi RE, Bertram L (2008) Systematic meta-analyses and field synopsis of genetic association studies in schizophrenia: the SzGene database. Nat Genet 40(7):827-34.
Alliey-Rodriguez N, Zhang D, Badner JA, Lahey BB, Zhang X, Dinwiddie S, Romanos B, Plenys N, Liu C, Gershon ES.Genome-wide association study of personality traits in bipolar patients. Psychiatr Genet. 2011 Aug;21(4):190-4. doi: 10.1097/YPG.0b013e3283457a31.

Ambrósio AM, Kennedy JL, Macciardi F, King N, Azevedo MH, Oliveira CR, Pato CN (2005) A linkage study between the GABAA beta2 and GABAA gamma2 subunit genes and major psychoses. CNS Spectr 10(1):57-61.

Anditsch M, Fasching P, Psota G, Rainer M, Walter A; Psychopharmaka Austria (2009).IFPA Interdisziplinäres Forum für Psychopharmako-Therapie im Alter (IFPA), ISBN: 978-3-200-01706-1

Angst J, Marneros A (2001) Bipolarity from ancient to modern times: conception, birth and rebirth. J Affect Disord 67(1-3):3-19.

Angst J (2002) Historical aspects of the dichotomy between manic-depressive disorders and schizophrenia.Schizophr Res 57(1):5-13.

Arai M, Itokawa M, Yamada K, Toyota T, Arai M, Haga S, Ujike H, Sora I, Ikeda K, Yoshikawa T (2004) Association of neural cell adhesion molecule 1 gene polymorphisms with bipolar affective disorder in Japanese individuals. Biol Psychiatry 55(8):804-10.

Archer SN, Robilliard DL, Skene DJ, Smits M, Williams A, Arendt J, von Schantz M (2003) A Length Polymorphism in the Circadian Clock Gene Per3 is Linked to Delayed Sleep Phase Syndrome and Extreme Diurnal Preference. Sleep 26(4):413-5

Arinami T, Itokawa M, Aoki J, Shibuya H, Ookubo Y, Iwawaki A, Ota K, Shimizu H, Hamaguchi H, Toru M (1996) Further association study on dopamine D2 receptor variant S311C in schizophrenia and affective disorders. Am J Med Genet 67(2):133-8.

Arinami T, Yamada N, Yamakawa-Kobayashi K, Hamaguchi H, Toru M (1997) Methylenetetrahydrofolate reductase variant and schizophrenia/depression. Am J Med Genet 74(5):526-8.

Arranz MJ, Erdmann J, Kirov G, Rietschel M, Sodhi M, Albus M, Ball D, Maier W, Davies N, Franzek E, Abusaad I, Weigelt B, Murray R, Shimron-Abarbanell D, Kerwin R, Propping P, Sham P, Nöthen MM, Collier DA (1997) 5-HT2A receptor and bipolar affective disorder: association studies in affected patients. Neurosci Lett 224(2):95-8.

Arts B, Simons CJ, Os Jv.Evidence for the impact of the CACNA1C risk allele rs1006737 on 2-year cognitive functioning in bipolar disorder. Psychiatr Genet. 2013 Feb;23(1):41-2. doi: 10.1097/YPG.0b013e328358641c.

Asherson P, Mant R, Williams N, Cardno A, Jones L, Murphy K, Collier DA, Nanko S, Craddock N, Morris S, Muir W, Blackwood B, McGuffin P, Owen MJ (1998) A study of chromosome 4p markers and dopamine D5 receptor gene in schizophrenia and bipolar disorder. Mol Psychiatry 3(4):310-20.

Askland K, Read C, Moore J (2009) Pathways-based analyses of whole-genome association study data in bipolar disorder reveal genes mediating ion channel activity and synaptic neurotransmission. Hum Genet 125:63-79

Aslund C, Leppert J, Comasco E, Nordquist N, Oreland L, Nilsson KW (2009) Impact of the interaction between the 5HTTLPR polymorphism and maltreatment on adolescent depression. A population-based study. Behav Genet 39(5):524-31. Epub 2009 Jul 7.

Athanasiu L, Mattingsdal M, Kähler AK, Brown A, Gustafsson O, Agartz I, Giegling I, Muglia P, Cichon S, Rietschel M, Pietiläinen OP, Peltonen L, Bramon E, Collier D, Clair DS, Sigurdsson E, Petursson H, Rujescu D, Melle I, Steen VM, Djurovic S, Andreassen OA.Gene variants associated with schizophrenia in a Norwegian genome-wide study are replicated in a large European cohort. J Psychiatr Res. 2010 Sep;44(12):748-53. doi: 10.1016/j.jpsychires.2010.02.002. Epub 2010 Feb 24.

Atz ME, Rollins B, Vawter MP (2007) NCAM1 association study of bipolar disorder and schizophrenia: polymorphisms and alternatively spliced isoforms lead to similarities and differences.Psychiatr Genet 17(2):55-67.

Avramopoulos D, Lasseter VK, Fallin MD, Wolyniec PS, McGrath JA, Nestadt G, Valle D, Pulver AE (2007) Stage II follow-up on a linkage scan for bipolar disorder in the Ashkenazim provides suggestive evidence for chromosome 12p and the GRIN2B gene. Genet Med 9(11):745-51. Abstract

B:

Bach AW, Lan NC, Johnson DL, Abell CW, Bembenek ME, Kwan SW, Seeburg PH, Shih JC (1988) cDNA cloning of human liver monoamine oxidase A and B: molecular basis of differences in enzymatic properties. Proc Natl Acad Sci USA 85:4934–4938

Badenhop RF, Moses MJ, Scimone A, Mitchell PB, Ewen KR, Rosso A, Donald JA, Adams LJ, Schofield PR (Badenhop) A genome screen of a large bipolar affective disorder pedigree supports evidence for a susceptibility locus on chromosome 13q. Mol Psychiatry 6(4):396-403.

Baekken PM, Skorpen F, Stordal E, Zwart JA, Hagen K (2008) Depression and anxiety in relation to catechol-O-methyltransferase Val158Met genotype in the general population: the Nord-Trøndelag Health Study (HUNT). BMC Psychiatry 8:48.

Bhakta SG, Zhang JP, Malhotra AK. The COMT Met158 allele and violence in schizophrenia: a meta-analysis. Schizophr Res. 2012 Sep;140(1-3):192-7. doi: 10.1016/j.schres.2012.06.026. Epub 2012 Jul 10.

Baltin J, Leist S, Odronitz F, Wollscheid HP, Baack M, Kapitza T, Schaarschmidt D, Knippers R (2006) DNA replication in protein extracts from human cells requires ORC and MCM proteins. J Biol Chem 281(18):12428-35. Epub 2006 Mar 13.

Bambico FR, Nguyen NT, Gobbi G (2009) Decline in serotonergic firing activity and desensitization of 5-HT1A autoreceptors after chronic unpredictable stress. Eur Neuropsychopharmacol 19(3):215-28.

Barden N, Harvey M, Gagné B, Shink E, Tremblay M, Raymond C, Labbé M, Villeneuve A, Rochette D, Bordeleau L, Stadler H, Holsboer F, Müller-Myhsok B (2006) Analysis of single nucleotide polymorphisms in genes in the chromosome 12Q24.31 region points to P2RX7 as a susceptibility gene to bipolar affective disorder. Am J Med Genet B Neuropsychiatr Genet 141B(4):374-82.

Barnett JH, Smoller JW, The genetics of bipolar disorder, Neuroscience (2009), doi: 10.1016/j. neuroscience.2009.03.080

Barrett TB, Emberton JE, Nievergelt CM, Liang SG, Hauger RL, Eskin E, Schork NJ, Kelsoe JR (2007) Further evidence for association of GRK3 to bipolar disorder suggests a second disease mutation.Psychiatr Genet 17(6):315-22 Abstract

Baron M, Risch N, Hamburger R, Mandel B, Kushner S, Newman M, Drumer D, Belmaker RH (1987) Genetic linkage between X-chromosome markers and bipolar affective illness. Nature 326(6110):289-92.

Baron M, Straub RE, Lehner T, Endicott J, Ott J, Gilliam TC, Lerer B (1994) Bipolar disorder and linkage to Xq28. Nat Genet 7(4):461-2.

Bass NJ, Datta SR, McQuillin A, Puri V, Choudhury K, Thirumalai S, Lawrence J, Quested D, Pimm J, Curtis D, Gurling HM (2009) Evidence for the association of the DAOA (G72) gene with schizophrenia and bipolar disorder but not for the association of the DAO gene with schizophrenia. Behav Brain Funct 5:28

Bhat RV, Budd Haeberlein SL, Avila J (2004) Glycogen synthase kinase 3: a drug target for CNS therapies. J Neurochem 89(6):1313-7.

Battersby S, Ogilvie AD, Smith CA, Blackwood DH, Muir WJ, Quinn JP, Fink G, Goodwin GM, Harmar AJ (1996) Structure of a variable number tandem repeat of the serotonin transporter gene and association with affective disorder. Psychiatr Genet 6(4):177-81. Abstract

Baysal BE, Willett-Brozick JE, Badner JA, Corona W, Ferrell RE, Nimgaonkar VL, Detera-Wadleigh SD (2002) A mannosyltransferase gene at 11q23 is disrupted by a translocation breakpoint that co-segregates with bipolar affective disorder in a small family. Neurogenetics 4(1):43-53.

Bauer M, Beaulieu S, Dunner DL, Lafer B, Kupka R (2008) Rapid cycling bipolar disorder – diagnostic concepts. Bipolar Disord 10(1 Pt 2):153-62.

Baum AE, Hamshere M, Green E, Cichon S, Rietschel M, Noethen MM, Craddock N, McMahon FJ (2008) Meta-analysis of two genome-wide association studies of bipolar disorder reveals important points of agreement. Mol Psychiatry 13(5):466-7. 1B

Baum AE, Akula N, Cabanero M, Cardona I, Corona W, Klemens B, Schulze TG, Cichon S, Rietschel M, Nöthen MM, Georgi A, Schumacher J, Schwarz M, Abou Jamra R, Höfels S, Propping P, Satagopan J, Detera-Wadleigh SD, Hardy J, McMahon FJ (2008) A genome-wide association study implicates diacylglycerol kinase eta (DGKH) and several other genes in the etiology of bipolar disorder. Mol Psychiatry 13(2):197-207. Epub 2007 May 8.

Baumer FM, Howe M, Gallelli K, Simeonova DI, Hallmayer J, Chang KD (2006) A pilot study of antidepressant-induced mania in pediatric bipolar disorder: Characteristics, risk factors, and the serotonin transporter gene. Biol Psychiatry 60(9):1005-12. Epub 2006 Aug 30.

Baune BT, Hohoff C, Berger K, Neumann A, Mortensen S, Roehrs T, Deckert J, Arolt V, Domschke K. (2008) Association of the COMT val158met variant with antidepressant treatment response in major depression. Neuropsychopharmacology 33(4):924-32.

Bellivier F, Henry C, Szöke A, Schürhoff F, Nosten-Bertrand M, Feingold J, Launay JM, Leboyer M, Laplanche JL (1998) Serotonin transporter gene polymorphisms in patients with unipolar or bipolar depression. Neurosci Lett 255(3):143-6.

Bellivier F, Leboyer M, Courtet P, Buresi C, Beaufils B, Samolyk D, Allilaire JF, Feingold J, Mallet J, Malafosse A (1998) Association between the tryptophan hydroxylase gene and manic-depressive illness. Arch Gen Psychiatry 55(1):33-7.

Bellivier F, Leroux M, Henry C, Rayah F, Rouillon F, Laplanche JL, Leboyer M (2002) Serotonin transporter gene polymorphism influences age at onset in patients with bipolar affective disorder. Neurosci Lett 334(1):17-20.

Belmonte Mahon, P, Pirooznia, M, Goes, FS, Seifuddin, F, Steele, J, Lee, PH, Huang, J, Hamshere, ML, Bipolar Genome Study (BiGS) Consortium, The Wellcome Trust Case Control Consortium Bipolar Disorder Group, Depaulo, JR, Jr, Kelsoe, JR, Rietschel, M, Nothen, M, Cichon, S, Gurling, H, Purcell, S, Smoller, JW, Craddock, N, Schulze, TG, McMahon, FJ, Potash, JB, Zandi, PP, 2011. Genome-wide association analysis of age at onset and psychotic symptoms in bipolar disorder. Am. J. Med. Genet. B. Neuropsychiatr. Genet. 156B, 370-378

Benazzi F, Akiskal HS (2006) Biphasic course in bipolar II outpatients: prevalence and clinical correlates of a cyclic pattern described by Baillarger and Falret in hospitalised patients in 1854. J Affect Disord 96(3):183-7.

Benedetti F, Serretti A, Colombo C, Campori E, Barbini B, di Bella D, Smeraldi E (1999) Influence of a functional polymorphism within the promoter of the serotonin transporter gene on the effects of total sleep deprivation in bipolar depression. Am J Psychiatry 156(9):1450-2.

Benedetti F, Serretti A, Colombo C, Barbini B, Lorenzi C, Campori E, Smeraldi E (2003) Influence of CLOCK gene polymorphism on circadian mood fluctuation and illness recurrence in bipolar depression. Am J Med Genet B Neuropsychiatr Genet 123B(1):23-6

Benedetti F, Dallaspezia S, Fulgosi MC, Lorenzi C, Serretti A, Barbini B, Colombo C, Smeraldi E (2007) Actimetric Evidence That CLOCK 3111 T/C SNP Influences Sleep and Activity Patterns in Patients Affected by Bipolar Depression. American Journal of Medical Genetics Part B (Neuropsychiatric Genetics) 144B:631–635

Benedetti F, Dallaspezia S, Colombo C, Pirovano A, Marino E, Smeraldi E (2008) A length polymorphism in the circadian clock gene Per3 influences age at onset of bipolar disorder. Neuroscience Letters 445:184-187

Benkert Otto, Hippius H: *Kompendium der Psychiatrischen Pharmakotherapie.* 8. Auflage, Springer, Berlin / Heilderberg, New York, NY 2011, ISBN 978-3-642-13043-4.

Berry N, Jobanputra V, Pal H (2003) Molecular genetics of schizophrenia: a critical review. J Psychiatry Neurosci 28(6):415-29.

Bet PM, Penninx BWJH, Bochdanovits Z, Uitterlinden AG, Beekman ATF, van Schoor NM, Deeg DJH, Hoogendijk WJG (2009) Glucocorticoid Receptor Gene Polymorphisms and Childhood Adversity Are Associated With Depression: New Evidence for a Gene–Environment Interaction. Am J Med Genet Part B 150B:660–669.

Binder DK, Scharfman H (2004) Brain-derived Neurotrophic Factor. Growth Factors 22 (3): 123-131

Binder EB, Bradley RG, Liu W, Epstein MP, Deveau TC, Mercer KB, Tang Y, Gillespie CF, Heim CM, Nemeroff CB, Schwartz AC, Cubells JF, Ressler KJ (2008) Association of FKBP5 polymorphisms and childhood abuse with risk of posttraumatic stress disorder symptoms in adults. JAMA 299(11):1291-305.

Birkett JT, Arranz MJ, Munro J, Osbourn S, Kerwin RW, Collier DA (2000) Association analysis of the 5-HT5A gene in depression, psychosis and antipsychotic response. Neuroreport 11(9):2017-20.

Bishara D, Taylor D (2009) Asenapine monotherapy in the acute treatment of both schizophrenia and bipolar I disorder. Neuropsychiatr Dis Treat 5:483-90. Epub 2009 Oct 12.

Black GC, Chen ZY, Craig IW, Powell JF (1991) Dinucleotide repeat polymorphism at the MAOA locus.Nucleic Acids Res 19:689

Blackwood DH, Fordyce A, Walker MT, St Clair DM, Porteous DJ, Muir WJ (2001) Schizophrenia and affective disorders – cosegregation with a translocation at chromosome 1q42 that directly disrupts brain-expressed genes: clinical and P300 findings in a family.Am J Hum Genet 69(2):428-33. Epub 2001 Jul 6.

Blairy S, Massat I, Staner L, Le Bon O, Van Gestel S, Van Broeckhoven C, Hilger C, Hentges F, Souery D, Mendlewicz J (2000) 5-HT2a receptor polymorphism gene in bipolar disorder and harm avoidance personality trait. Am J Med Genet 96(3):360-4.

Bloom FE, Morales M (1998) The central 5-HT3 receptor in CNS disorders. Neurochem Res 23(5):653-9.

Bode L, Reckwald P, Severus WE, Stoyloff R, Ferszt R, Dietrich DE, Ludwig H (2001) Borna disease virus-specific circulating immune complexes, antigenemia, and free antibodies-the key marker triplet determining infection and prevailing in severe mood disorders. Mol Psychiatry 6(4):481-91.

Bocchetta A, Piccardi MP, Palmas MA, Chillotti C, Oi A, Del Zompo M (1999) Family-based association study between bipolar disorder and DRD2, DRD4, DAT, and SERT in Sardinia. Am J Med Genet 88(5):522-6.

Bogdanović O, Veenstra GJ (2009) DNA methylation and methyl-CpG binding proteins: developmental requirements and function. Chromosoma 118(5): 549-65.

Bonhomme N, De Deurwaerdere P, Le Moal M, Spampinato U (1995) Evidence for 5-HT4 receptor subtype involvement in the enhancement of striatal dopamine release induced by serotonin: a microdialysis study in the halothane-anesthetized rat. Neuropharmacology 34: 269-279.

Bonnier B, Gorwood P, Hamon M, Sarfati Y, Boni C, Hardy-Bayle MC (2002) Association of 5-HT(2A) receptor gene polymorphism with major affective disorders: the case of a subgroup of bipolar disorder with low suicide risk. Biol Psychiatry 51(9):762-5.

Bradley RG, Binder EB, Epstein MP, Tang Y, Nair HP, Liu W, Gillespie CF, Berg T, Evces M, Newport DJ, Stowe ZN, Heim CM, Nemeroff CB, Schwartz A, Cubells JF, Ressler KJ (2008) Influence of Child Abuse on Adult Depression: Moderation by the Corticotropin-Releasing Hormone Receptor Gene. Arch Gen Psychiatry. Author manuscript; available in PMC 2008 July 7. PMCID: PMC2443704

Breen G, Prata D, Osborne S, Munro J, Sinclair M, Li T, Staddon S, Dempster D, Sainz R, Arroyo B, Kerwin RW, St Clair D, Collier D (2006) Association of the dysbindin gene with bipolar affective disorder. Am J Psychiatry 163(9):1636-8.

Brisch R, Bernstein HG, Krell D, Dobrowolny H, Bielau H, Steiner J, Gos T, Funke S, Stauch R, Knüppel S, Bogerts B (2009) Dopamine-glutamate abnormalities in the frontal cortex associated with the catechol-O-methyltransferase (COMT) in schizophrenia. Brain Res 1269:166-75. Epub 2009 Mar 4.

Brown GW, Harris TO (2008) Depression and the serotonin transporter 5-HTTLPR polymorphism: a review and a hypothesis concerning gene-environment interaction. J Affect Disord 111(1):1-12. Epub 2008 Jun 4.

Brueckner F, Armache KJ, Cheung A, Damsma GE, Kettenberger H, Lehmann E, Sydow J, Cramer P (2009) Structure-function studies of the RNA polymerase II elongation complex. Acta Crystallogr D Biol Crystallogr 65:112-20.

Brunner HG, Nelen MR, van Zandvoort P, Abeling NG, van Gennip AH, Wolters EC, Kuiper MA, Ropers HH, van Oost BA (1993) X-linked borderline mental retardation with prominent behavioral disturbance: phenotype, genetic localization, and evidence for disturbed monoamine metabolism. Am J Hum Genet 52(6):1032–1039.

Bunger MK, Wilsbacher LD, Moran SM, Clendenin C, Radcliffe LA, Hogenesch JB, Simon MC, Takahashi JS, Bradfield CA (2000) Mop3 is an essential component of the master circadian pacemaker in mammals. Cell 103(7):1009-17.

Burdick KE, Funke B, Goldberg JF, Bates JA, Jaeger J, Kucherlapati R, Malhotra AK (2007) COMT genotype increases risk for bipolar I disorder and influences neurocognitive performance. Bipolar Disord 9(4):370-6.

Burmeister M, McInnis MG, Zöllner S (2008) Psychiatric genetics: progress amid controversy. Nat Rev Genet 9(7):527-40.

Buselmaier Tariverdian (2004) Humangenetik. 3.Auflage. Springer Verlag.

C:

Campos SB, Miranda DM, Souza BR, Pereira PA, Neves FS, Bicalho MA, Melillo PH, Tramontina J, Kapczinski F, Romano-Silva MA, Correa H. Association of polymorphisms of the tryptophan hydroxylase 2 gene with risk for bipolar disorder or suicidal behavior.J Psychiatr Res. 2010 Apr;44(5):271-4. doi: 10.1016/j.jpsychires.2009.09.007. Epub 2009 Oct 1.

Campos SB, Miranda DM, Souza BR, Pereira PA, Neves FS, Tramontina J, Kapczinski F, Romano-Silva MA, Correa H.Association study of tryptophan hydroxylase 2 gene polymorphisms in bipolar disorder patients with panic disorder comorbidity. Psychiatr Genet. 2011 Apr; 21(2):106-11. doi: 10.1097/YPG.0b013e328341a3a8.

Cannas A, Spissu A, Floris GL, Congia S, Saddi MV, Melis M, Mascia MM, Pinna F, Tuveri A, Solla P, Milia A, Giagheddu M, Tacconi P (2002) Bipolar affective disorder and Parkinson's disease: a rare, insidious and often unrecognized association. Neurol Sci 2:S67-8.

Cannon DM, Klaver JM, Peck SA, Rallis-Voak D, Erickson K, Drevets WC (2009) Dopamine type-1 receptor binding in major depressive disorder assessed using positron emission tomography and [11C]NNC-112. Neuropsychopharmacology 34(5):1277-87.

Cardno Alastair G, Marshall JA, Bina Coid, PhD; Alison M Macdonald, PhD; Tracy R Ribchester, BSc; Nadia J Davies, MB, MRCPsych; Piero Venturi, MD; Lisa A Jones, BSc; Shôn W Lewis, MD, FRCPsych; Pak C Sham, MB,

MRCPsych; Irving I Gottesman, PhD; Anne E Farmer, MD, MRCPsych; Peter McGuffin, MB, PhD, FRCPsych; Adrianne M Reveley, MB, MRCPsych; Robin M Murray, MD, FRCPsych, DSc (1999) Heritability Estimates for Psychotic Disorders-The Maudsley Twin Psychosis Series. Arch Gen Psychiatry 56:162-168

Carlson C, Papolos D, Pandita RK, Faedda GL, Veit S, Goldberg R, Shprintzen R, Kucherlapati R and Morrow B (1997) Molecular Analysis of Velo-Cardio-Facial Syndrome Patients with Psychiatric Disorders. Am. J. Hum. Genet 60:851-859

Carter CJ (2007) EIF2B and Oligodendrocyte Survival: Where Nature and Nurture Meet in Bipolar Disorder and Schizophrenia? Schizophr Bull 33(6): 1343-1353.

Carter R, Drouin G (2009) Structural differentiation of the three eukaryotic RNA polymerases. Genomics 94(6):388-96.

Casamassima F, Huang J, Fava M, Sachs GS, Smoller JW, Cassano GB, Lattanzi L, Fagerness J, Stange JP, Perlis RH (2010) Phenotypic effects of a bipolar liability gene among individuals with major depressive disorder. Am J Med Genet B Neuropsychiatr Genet 153B(1):303-9.

Cases O, Seif I, Grimsby J, Gaspar P, Chen K, Pournin S, Müller U, Aguet M, Babinet C, Shih JC, et al. (1995) Aggressive behavior and altered amounts of brain serotonin and norepinephrine in mice lacking MAOA. Science 268(5218):1763-6

Caspi A, McClay J, Moffitt TE, Mill J, Martin J, Craig IW, et al. (2002) Role of genotype in the cycle of violence in maltreated children. Science 297:851-4.

Caspi A, Sugden K, Moffitt TE, Taylor A, Craig IW, Harrington H, McClay J, Mill J, Martin J, Braithwaite A, Poulton R (2003) Influence of life stress on depression: moderation by a polymorphism in the 5-HTT gene. Science 301(5631):386-9.

Cassidy F, Zhao C, Badger J, Claffey E, Dobrin S, Roche S, McKeon P (2007) Genome-wide scan of bipolar disorder and investigation of population stratification effects on linkage: support for susceptibility loci at 4q21, 7q36, 9p21, 12q24, 14q24, and 16p13.Am J Med Genet B Neuropsychiatr Genet 144B(6):791-801.

Ceulemans S, De Zutter S, Heyrman L, Norrback KF, Nordin A, Nilsson LG, Adolfsson R, Del-Favero J, Claes S. Evidence for the involvement of the glucocorticoid receptor gene in bipolar disorder in an isolated northern Swedish population.Bipolar Disord. 2011 Nov-Dec;13(7-8):614-23. doi: 10.1111/j.1399-5618.2011.00960.x.

Cermakian N, Boivin DB (2003) A molecular perspective of human circadian rhythm disorders. Brain Research Reviews 42: 204-220

Chang CC, Lu RB, Ma KH, Chang HA, Chen CL, Huang CC, Lin WW, Huang SY (2007) Association study of the norepinephrine transporter gene polymorphisms and bipolar disorder in Han Chinese population. World J Biol Psychiatry 8(3):188-95.Abstract

Chang YC, Rapoport SI, Rao JS (2009) Chronic Administration of Mood Stabilizers Upregulates BDNF and Bcl-2 Expression Levels in Rat Frontal Cortex. Neurochem Res 34(3):536-541

Chapman RD, Palancade B, Lang A, Bensaude O, Eick D (2004) The last CTD repeat of the mammalian RNA polymerase II large subunit is important for its stability. Nucleic Acids Res 32(1):35-44.

Chen Z, Manley JL (2003) Core promoter elements and TAFs contribute to the diversity of transcriptional activation in vertebrates.Mol Cell Biol 23(20): 7350-62.

Chen K, Holschneider DP, Wu W, Rebrin I, Shih JC (2004) Spontaneous Point Mutation Produces Monoamine Oxidase A/B Knock-out Mice with Greatly Elevated Monoamines and Anxiety-like Behavior. J Biol Chem 279(38): 39645-52

Chen S, de Vries MA, Bell SP (2007) Orc6 is required for dynamic recruitment of Cdt1 during repeated Mcm2-7 loading.Genes Dev 21(22):2897-907.

Chen C, Glatt SJ,Tsuang MT (2008) The tryptophan hydroxylase gene influences risk for bipolar disorder but not major depressive disorder: results of meta-analyses. Bipolar Disord 10(7):816-21.

Chen L, Lawlor DA, Lewis SJ, Yuan W, Abdollahi MR, Timpson NJ, Day IN, Ebrahim S, Smith GD, Shugart YY (2008) Genetic association study of BDNF in depression: finding from two cohort studies and a meta-analysis. Am J Med Genet B Neuropsychiatr Genet 147B(6):814-21.

Chen DT, Jiang X, Akula N, Shugart YY, Wendland JR, Steele CJ, Kassem L, Park JH, Chatterjee N, Jamain S, Cheng A, Leboyer M, Muglia P, Schulze TG, Cichon S, Nöthen MM, Rietschel M; BiGS, McMahon FJ.Genome-wide association study meta-analysis of European and Asian-ancestry samples identifies three novel loci associated with bipolar disorder. Mol Psychiatry. 2011 Dec 20. doi: 10.1038/mp.2011.157.

Chien YL, Liu CM, Fann CS, Liu YL, Hwu HG (2009) Association of the 3' region of COMT with schizophrenia in Taiwan. J Formos Med Assoc 108(4):301-9.

Choi KY, Yoon HK, Kim YK.Association between Serotonin-Related Polymorphisms in 5HT2A, TPH1, TPH2 Genes and Bipolar Disorder in Korean Population. Psychiatry Investig. 2010 Mar; 7(1):60-7. doi: 10.4306/pi. 2010.7.1.60. Epub 2010 Mar 3.

Chou YH, Wang SJ, Lin CL, Mao WC, Lee SM, Liao MH.Decreased brain serotonin transporter binding in the euthymic state of bipolar I but not bipolar II disorder: a SPECT study. Bipolar Disord. 2010 May;12(3):312-8. doi: 10.1111/j.1399-5618.2010.00800.x.

Chorbov VM, Lobos EA, Todorov AA, Heath AC, Botteron KN, Todd RD (2007) Relationship of 5-HTTLPR Genotypes and Depression Risk in the Presence of Trauma in a Female Twin Sample. Am J Med Genet Part B 144B:830-833.

Chotai J, Serretti A, Lattuada E, Lorenzi C, Lilli R (2003) Gene-environment interaction in psychiatric disorders as indicated by season of birth variations in tryptophan hydroxylase (TPH), serotonin transporter (5-HTTLPR) and dopamine receptor (DRD4) gene polymorphisms. Psychiatry Res 119(1-2):99-111.

Chotai J, Serretti A, Lorenzi C (2005) Interaction between the tryptophan hydroxylase gene and the serotonin transporter gene in schizophrenia but not in bipolar or unipolar affective disorders. Neuropsychobiology 51(1):3-9.

Christensen EM, Larsen JK, Gjerris A, Peacock L, Jacobi M, Hassenbalch E (2008) Climatic factors and bipolar affective disorder. Nord J Psychiatry 62(1):55-8. Abstract

Cichon S, Winge I, Mattheisen M, Georgi A, Karpushova A, Freudenberg J, Freudenberg-Hua Y, Babadjanova G, Van Den Bogaert A, Abramova LI, Kapiletti S, Knappskog PM, McKinney J, Maier W, Jamra RA, Schulze TG, Schumacher J, Propping P, Rietschel M, Haavik J, Nöthen MM. Brain-specific tryptophan hydroxylase 2 (TPH2): a functional Pro206Ser substitution and variation in the 5'-region are associated with bipolar affective disorder. Hum Mol Genet. 2008 Jan 1;17(1):87-97. Epub 2007 Sep 27.

Cichon S, Mühleisen TW, Degenhardt FA, Mattheisen M, Miró X, Strohmaier J, Steffens M, Meesters C, Herms S, Weingarten M, Priebe L, Haenisch B, Alexander M, Vollmer J, Breuer R, Schmäl C, Tessmann P, Moebus S, Wichmann HE, Schreiber S, Müller-Myhsok B, Lucae S, Jamain S, Leboyer M, Bellivier F, Etain B, Henry C, Kahn JP, Heath S; Bipolar Disorder Genome Study (BiGS) Consortium, Hamshere M, O'Donovan MC, Owen MJ, Craddock N, Schwarz M, Vedder H, Kammerer-Ciernioch J, Reif A, Sasse J, Bauer M, Hautzinger M, Wright A, Mitchell PB, Schofield PR, Montgomery GW, Medland SE, Gordon SD, Martin NG, Gustafsson O, Andreassen O, Djurovic S, Sigurdsson E, Steinberg S, Stefansson H, Stefansson K, Kapur-Pojskic L, Oruc L, Rivas F, Mayoral F, Chuchalin A, Babadjanova G, Tiganov AS, Pantelejeva G, Abramova LI, Grigoroiu-Serbanescu M, Diaconu CC, Czerski PM, Hauser J, Zimmer A, Lathrop M, Schulze TG, Wienker TF, Schumacher J, Maier W, Propping P, Rietschel M, Nöthen MM. Genome-wide association study identifies genetic variation in neurocan as a susceptibility factor for bipolar disorder.Am J Hum Genet. 2011 Mar 11;88(3):372-81. Epub 2011 Feb 25. Erratum in: Am J Hum Genet. 2011 Mar 11;88(3):396.

Chiesa A, Crisafulli C, Porcelli S, Balzarro B, Han C, Patkar AA, Lee SJ, Park MH, Pae CU, Serretti A.Case-control association study of GRIA1, GRIA2 and GRIA4 polymorphisms in bipolar disorder. Int J Psychiatry Clin Pract. 2012 Mar;16(1):18-26. doi: 10.3109/13651501.2011.617459. Epub 2011 Oct 31.

Collier DA, Arranz MJ, Sham P, Battersby S, Vallada H, Gill P, Aitchison KJ, Sodhi M, Li T, Roberts GW, Smith B, Morton J, Murray RM, Smith D, Kirov G (1996) The serotonin transporter is a potential susceptibility factor for bipolar affective disorder. Neuroreport 7(10):1675-9 Abstract

Conrad DF, Pinto D, Redon R, Feuk L, Gokcumen O, Zhang Y, Aerts J, Andrews TD, Barnes C, Campbell P, Fitzgerald T, Hu M, Ihm CH, Kristiansson K, Macarthur DG, Macdonald JR, Onyiah I, Pang AW, Robson S, Stirrups K, Valsesia A, Walter K, Wei J; The Wellcome Trust Case Control Consortium, Tyler-Smith C, Carter NP, Lee C, Scherer SW, Hurles ME (2009) Origins and functional impact of copy number variation in the human genome. Nature

Comasco E, Sylvén SM, Papadopoulos FC, Sundström-Poromaa I, Oreland L, Skalkidou A. Psychiatr Genet. 2011 Feb; 21(1):19-28. doi: 10.1097/ YPG.0b013e328341a3c1.Postpartum depression symptoms: a case-control study on monoaminergic functional polymorphisms and environmental stressors. Psychiatr Genet. 2011 Feb;21(1):19-28. doi: 10.1097/YPG.0b013e3 28341a3c1.

Cordeiro Q, Talkowski ME, Chowdari KV, Wood J, Nimgaonkar V, Vallada H (2005) Association and linkage analysis of RGS4 polymorphisms with schizophrenia and bipolar disorder in Brazil.Genes Brain Behav 4(1):45-50.

Cordeiro Q, Siqueira-Roberto J, Zung S, Vallada H. Association between the DRD2-141C Insertion/Deletion polymorphism and schizophrenia.Arq Neuropsiquiatr. 2009 Jun;67(2A):191-4.

Corvin A, Donohoe G, Nangle JM, Schwaiger S, Morris D, Gill M. A dysbindin risk haplotype associated with less severe manic-type symptoms in psychosis.Neurosci Lett. 2008 Jan 31;431(2):146-9. Epub 2007 Dec 4.

Coryell W, Leon AC, Turvey C, Akiskal HS, Mueller T, Endicott J (2001) The significance of psychotic features in manic episodes: a report from the NIMH collaborative study. J Affect Disord 67(1-3):79-88.

Correa H, De Marco L, Boson W, Viana MM, Lima VF, Campi-Azevedo AC, Noronha JC, Guatimosim C, Romano-Silva MA (2002) Analysis of T102C 5HT2A polymorphism in Brazilian psychiatric inpatients: relationship with suicidal behavior. Cell Mol Neurobiol 22(5-6):813-7.

Cosgrove VE, Miklowitz DJ, Rhee SH, Hawkey C, Corley R, Haberstick B, Smolen A. Association between 5HTT, DAT1, and DRD4 and bipolar disorder in youth. Psychiatr Genet. 2012 Dec;22(6):304. doi: 10.1097/YPG.0b013e3 283539517. No abstract available.

Coyle N, Jones I, Robertson E, Lendon C, Craddock N (2000) Variation at the serotonin transporter gene influences susceptibility to bipolar affective puerperal psychosis. Lancet 356(9240):1490-1.

Craddock N, Dawson E, Burge S, Parfitt L, Mant B, Roberts Q, Daniels J, Gill M, McGuffin P, Powell J, et al. (1993)The gene for Darier's disease maps to chromosome 12q23-q24.1.Hum Mol Genet 2(11):1941-3. Erratum in: Hum Mol Genet 1993 Dec;2(12):2214.

Craddock N, Daniels J, Roberts E, Rees M, McGuffin P, Owen MJ (1995) No evidence for allelic association between bipolar disorder and monoamine oxidase A gene polymorphisms. Am J Med Genet 60(4):322-4.

Craddock N, Owen MJ (1996) Candidate gene association studies in psychiatric genetics: a SERTain future? Mol Psychiatry 1(6):434-6. Abstract

Craddock N, Lendon C (1999) Chromosome Workshop: chromosomes 11, 14, and 15. Am J Med Genet 88(3):244-54.

Craddock N, Davé S, Greening J (2001) Association studies of bipolar disorder.Bipolar Disord 3(6):284-98.

Craddock N, O'Donovan MC, Owen MJ (2009) Psychosis genetics: modeling the relationship between schizophrenia, bipolar disorder, and mixed (or "schizoaffective") psychoses. Schizophr Bull 35(3):482-90.

Craddock N, O'Donovan MC, Owen MJ (2006) Genes for Schizophrenia and Bipolar Disorder? Implications for Psychiatric Nosology. Schizophr Bull 32(1): 9-16.

Craddock N, Sklar P (2009) Genetics of bipolar disorder: successful start to a long journey. Trends Genet 25(2):99-105. Epub 2009 Jan 12.

CRICK FH, BARNETT L, BRENNER S, WATTS-TOBIN RJ (1961) General nature of the genetic code for proteins.Nature 192:1227-32.

Cronholm B, Asberg M, Montgomery S, Schalling D (1977) Suicidal behaviour syndrome with low CSF 5-HIAA.Br Med J 1(6063):776.

Crowe RR, Vieland V (1999) Report of the Chromosome 5 Workshop of the Sixth World Congress on Psychiatric Genetics. Am J Med Genet 88(3):229-32.

Cunha AB, Frey BN, Andreazza AC, Goi JD, Rosa AR, Gonçalves CA, Santin A, Kapczinski F (2006) Serum brain-derived neurotrophic factor is decreased in bipolar disorder during depressive and manic episodes. Neurosci Lett. 398(3):215-9. Epub 2006 Feb 9.

Cusin C, Serretti A, Lattuada E, Lilli R, Lorenzi C, Mandelli L, Pisati E, Smeraldi E (2001) Influence of 5-HTTLPR and TPH variants on illness time course in mood disorders. J Psychiatr Res. 35(4):217-23.

D:

Dallaspezia S, Lorenzi C, Pirovano A, Colombo C, Smeraldi E, Benedetti F. Circadian clock gene Per3 variants influence the postpartum onset of bipolar disorder. Eur Psychiatry. 2011 Apr;26(3):138-40. doi: 10.1016/j.eurpsy. 2010.11.009

Dalvie S, Horn N, Nossek C, van der Merwe L, Stein DJ, Ramesar R.Psychosis and relapse in bipolar disorder are related to GRM3, DAOA, and GRIN2B genotype. Afr J Psychiatry (Johannesbg). 2010 Sep;13(4):297-301.

Dawson E, Parfitt E, Roberts Q, Daniels J, Lim L, Sham P, Nöthen M, Propping P, Lanczik M, Maier W, et al. (1995) Linkage studies of bipolar disorder in the region of the Darier's disease gene on chromosome 12q23-24.1. Am J Med Genet 60(2):94-102. Abstract

Davies PA, Pistis M, Hanna MC, Peters JA, Lambert JJ, Hales TG, Kirkness EF (1999) The 5-HT3B subunit is a major determinant of serotonin-receptor function. Nature 397(6717):359-63.

Dean B, Digney A, Sundram S, Thomas E, Scarr E (2008) Plasma apolipoprotein E is decreased in schizophrenia spectrum and bipolar disorder.Psychiatry Res 158(1):75-8.

De bruyn A, Mendelbaum K, Sandkuijl LA, Delvenne V, Hirsch D, Staner L, Mendlewicz J, Van Broeckhoven C (1994) Nonlinkage of bipolar illness to tyrosine hydroxylase, tyrosinase, and D2 and D4 dopamine receptor genes on chromosome 11. Am J Psychiatry 151(1):102-6.

DeBruyne JP, Weaver DR, Reppert SM (2007) CLOCK and NPAS2 have overlapping roles in the suprachiasmatic circadian clock. Nat Neurosci 10(5):543-5.

Dedman A, McQuillin A, Kandaswamy R, Sharp S, Anjorin A, Gurling H. Sequencing of the ANKYRIN 3 gene (ANK3) encoding ankyrin G in bipolar disorder reveals a non-conservative amino acid change in a short isoform of ankyrin G. Am J Med Genet B Neuropsychiatr Genet. 2012 Apr; 159B(3): 328-35. doi: 10.1002/ajmg.b.32030. Epub 2012 Feb 10.

Degn B, Lundorf MD, Wang A, Vang M, Mors O, Kruse TA, Ewald H (2001) Further evidence for a bipolar risk gene on chromosome 12q24 suggested by investigation of haplotype sharing and allelic association in patients from the Faroe Islands. Mol Psychiatry. 2001 Jul; 6(4):450-5. Mol Psychiatry 6(4):450-5.

De Luca V, Tharmalingam S, King N, Strauss J, Bulgin N, Kennedy JL (2005) Association study of a novel functional polymorphism of the serotonin transporter gene in bipolar disorder and suicidal behaviour. Psychopharmacology (Berl). 182(1):128-31.

De Luca V, Strauss J, Semeralul M, Huang S, Li PP, Warsh JJ, Kennedy LJ, Wong HCA (2008) Analysis of BDNF Val66Met allele-specific mRNA levels in bipolar disorder. Neuroscience letters 441:229-232

De Luca V, Likhodi O, Kennedy JL, Wong AH (2007) Differential expression and parent-of-origin effect of the 5-HT2A receptor gene C102T polymorphism: analysis of suicidality in schizophrenia and bipolar disorder. Am J Med Genet B Neuropsychiatr Genet.144B(3):370-4.
De Luca V, Likhodi O, Kennedy JL, Wong AHC (2007) Parent-of-origin effect and genomic imprinting of the HTR2A receptor gene T102C polymorphism in psychosis. Psychiatry Research 151:243–248
Dempster EL, Mill J, Craig IW, Collier DA (2006) The quantification of COMT mRNA in post mortem cerebellum tissue: diagnosis, genotype, methylation and expression. BMC Med Genet 7:10.
Del Zompo M, De Luca V, Severino G, Ni X, Mulas S, Congiu D, Piccardi MP, Kennedy JL (2007) Haplotype association study between DRD1 gene and bipolar type I affective disorder in two samples from Canada and Sardinia. Am J Med Genet B Neuropsychiatr Genet 144B(2):237-41.
De Oliveira GS, Ceresér KM, Fernandes BS, Kauer-Sant'Anna M, Fries GR, Stertz L, Aguiar B, Pfaffenseller B, Kapczinski F. Decreased brain-derived neurotrophic factor in medicated and drug-free bipolar patients. J Psychiatr Res. 2009 Sep;43(14):1171-4. Epub 2009 May 26. Abstract
De Abreu LN, Lafer B, Baca-Garcia E, Oquendo MA (2009) Suicidal ideation and suicide attempts in bipolar disorder type I: an update for the clinician. Rev Bras Psiquiatr 31(3):271-80.
Derry JMJ, Lan NC, Shihl JC, Barnard EA and Barnard PJ (1989) Localization of monoamine oxidase A and B genes on the mouse X chromosome. Nucleic Acids Research 17(20):8403.
Desan PH, Oren DA, Malison R, Price LH, Rosenbaum J, Smoller J, Charney DS, Gelernter J (2000) Genetic Polymorphism at the CLOCK Gene Locus and Major Depression. American Journal of Medical Genetics (Neuropsychiatric Genetics) 96:418–421
DGBS e.V. und DGPPN e.V.: S3-Leitlinie zur Diagnostik und Therapie Bipolarer Störungen. Langversion, 2012
Detera-Wadleigh SD, Badner JA, Berrettini WH, Yoshikawa T, Goldin LR, Turner G, Rollins DY, Moses T, Sanders AR, Karkera JD, Esterling LE, Zeng J, Ferraro TN, Guroff JJ, Kazuba D, Maxwell ME, Nurnberger JI Jr, Gershon ES (1999) A high-density genome scan detects evidence for a bipolar-disorder susceptibility locus on 13q32 and other potential loci on 1q32 and 18p11.2. Proc Natl Acad Sci U S A. 96(10):5604-9.
Dick DM, Foroud T, Flury L, Bowman ES, Miller MJ, Rau NL, Moe PR, Samavedy N, El-Mallakh R, Manji H, Glitz DA, Meyer ET, Smiley C, Hahn R, Widmark C, McKinney R, Sutton L, Ballas C, Grice D, Berrettini W, Byerley W, Coryell W, DePaulo R, MacKinnon DF, Gershon ES, Kelsoe JR, McMa-

hon FJ, McInnis M, Murphy DL, Reich T, Scheftner W, Nurnberger JI Jr (2003) Genomewide linkage analyses of bipolar disorder: a new sample of 250 pedigrees from the National Institute of Mental Health Genetics Initiative. Am J Hum Genet.73(1):107-14.

Dickerson FB, Boronow JJ, Stallings C, Origoni AE, Cole S, Leister F, Krivogorsky B, Yolken RH (2006) The catechol O-methyltransferase Val158Met polymorphism and herpes simplex virus type 1 infection are risk factors for cognitive impairment in bipolar disorder: additive gene-environmental effects in a complex human psychiatric disorder. Bipolar Disord. 8(2): 124-32.

Dimitrova A, Georgieva L, Nikolov I, Poriazova N, Krastev S, Toncheva D, Owen MJ, Kirov G (2002) Major psychiatric disorders and the serotonin transporter gene (SLC6A4): family-based association studies. Psychiatr Genet. 2002 Sep;12(3):137-41.Abstract

Digney A, Keriakous D, Scarr E, Thomas E, Dean B (2005) Differential changes in apolipoprotein E in schizophrenia and bipolar I disorder. Biol Psychiatry.57(7):711-5.

Djurovic S, Gustafsson O, Mattingsdal M, Athanasiu L, Bjella T, Tesli M, Agartz I, Lorentzen S, Melle I, Morken G, Andreassen OA. A genome-wide association study of bipolar disorder in Norwegian individuals, followed by replication in Icelandic sample. J Affect Disord. 2010 Oct;126(1-2):312-6. Epub 2010 May 7.

Dmitrzak-Weglarz M, Rybakowski JK, Slopien A, Czerski PM, Leszczynska-Rodziewicz A, Kapelski P, Kaczmarkiewicz-Fass M, Hauser J (2006) Dopamine receptor D1 gene -48A/G polymorphism is associated with bipolar illness but not with schizophrenia in a Polish population. Neuropsychobiology. 53(1):46-50.

Domínguez E, Loza MI, Padín F, Gesteira A, Paz E, Páramo M, Brenlla J, Pumar E, Iglesias F, Cibeira A, Castro M, Caruncho H, Carracedo A, Costas J (2007) Extensive linkage disequilibrium mapping at HTR2A and DRD3 for schizophrenia susceptibility genes in the Galician population. Schizophr Res 90(1-3):123-9.

Dong C, Wong ML, Licinio J (2009) Sequence variations of ABCB1, SLC6A2, SLC6A3, SLC6A4, CREB1, CRHR1 and NTRK2: association with major depression and antidepressant response in Mexican-Americans. Mol Psychiatry 14(12):1105-18.

Duan J, Martinez M, Sanders AR, Hou C, Burrell GJ, Krasner AJ, Schwartz DB, Gejman PV (2007) DTNBP1 (Dystrobrevin binding protein 1) and schizophrenia: association evidence in the 3' end of the gene. Hum Hered 64(2):97-106.

Duan X, Chang JH, Ge S, Faulkner RL, Kim JY, Kitabatake Y, Liu XB, Yang CH, Jordan JD, Ma DK, Liu CY, Ganesan S, Cheng HJ, Ming GL, Lu B, Song H (2007 b) Disrupted-In-Schizophrenia 1 regulates integration of newly generated neurons in the adult brain.Cell 130(6):1146-58.

Dubertret C, Hanoun N, Adès J, Hamon M, Gorwood P (2004) Family-based association study of the serotonin-6 receptor gene (C267T polymorphism) in schizophrenia. Am J Med Genet B Neuropsychiatr Genet 126B(1):10-5.

E:

Engel GL (1978) The biopsychosocial model and the education of health professionals. Ann N Y Acad Sci 310:169-87.

Eastwood SL, Harrison PJ (2008) Decreased mRNA expression of netrin-G1 and netrin-G2 in the temporal lobe in schizophrenia and bipolar disorder. Neuropsychopharmacology 33(4):933-45.

Ebisawa T, Uchiyama M, Kajimura N, Mishima K, Kamei Y, Katoh M, Watanabe T, Sekimoto M, Shibui K, Kim K, Kudo Y, Ozeki Y, Sugishita M, Toyoshima R, Inoue Y, Yamada N, Nagase T, Ozaki N, Ohara O, Ishida N, Okawa M, Takahashi K, Yamauchi T (2001) Association of structural polymorphisms in the human period3 gene with delayed sleep phase syndrome. EMBO Rep 2(4):342-6

Eison AS, Mullins UL.Regulation of central 5-HT2A receptors: a review of in vivo studies. Behav Brain Res. 1996;73(1-2):177-81.

Engel G L (1977) The need for a new medical model : a challenge for biomedicine. Science 196: 129- 136

Egeland et al. (1987) Bipolar affective disorders linked to DNA markers on chromosome 11. Nature 325: 788-787

Ekholm JM, Pekkarinen P, Pajukanta P, Kieseppä T, Partonen T, Paunio T, Varilo T, Perola M, Lönnqvist J, Peltonen L (2002) Bipolar disorder susceptibility region on Xq24-q27.1 in Finnish families. Mol Psychiatry 7(5):453-9.

Ekholm JM, Kieseppä T, Hiekkalinna T, Partonen T, Paunio T, Perola M, Ekelund J, Lönnqvist J, Pekkarinen-Ijäs P, Peltonen L (2003) Evidence of susceptibility loci on 4q32 and 16p12 for bipolar disorder. Hum Mol Genet 12(15):1907-15.

Eley TC, Sugden K, Corsico A, Gregory AM, Sham P, McGuffin P, Plomin R, Craig IW (2004) Gene-environment interaction analysis of serotonin system markers with adolescent depression. Mol Psychiatry 9(10):908-15.

Elvidge G, Jones I, McCandless F, Asherson P, Owen MJ, Craddock N (2001) Allelic variation of a BalI polymorphism in the DRD3 gene does not influence susceptibility to bipolar disorder: results of analysis and meta-analysis. Am J Med Genet 105(4):307-11.

Emilien G, Maloteaux JM, Geurts M, Hoogenberg K, Cragg S (1999) Dopamine receptors – physiological understanding to therapeutic intervention potential. Pharmacol Ther 84(2):133-56.

Erk S, Meyer-Lindenberg A, Schnell K, Opitz von Boberfeld C, Esslinger C, Kirsch P, Grimm O, Arnold C, Haddad L, Witt SH, Cichon S, Nöthen MM, Rietschel M, Walter H. Brain function in carriers of a genome-wide supported bipolar disorder variant. Arch Gen Psychiatry. 2010 Aug; 67(8):803-11. doi: 10.1001/archgenpsychiatry.2010.94.

Etain B, Rousseva A, Roy I, Henry C, Malafosse A, Buresi C, Preisig M, Rayah F, Leboyer M, Bellivier F (2004) Lack of association between 5HT2A receptor gene haplotype, bipolar disorder and its clinical subtypes in a West European sample. Am J Med Genet B Neuropsychiatr Genet129B(1):29-33.

Etain B, Mathieu F, Rietschel M, Maier W, Albus M, McKeon P, Roche S, Kealey C, Blackwood D, Muir W, Bellivier F, Henry C, Dina C, Gallina S, Gurling H, Malafosse A, Preisig M, Ferrero F, Cichon S, Schumacher J, Ohlraun S, Borrmann-Hassenbach M, Propping P, Abou Jamra R, Schulze TG, Marusic A, Dernovsek ZM, Giros B, Bourgeron T, Lemainque A, Bacq D, Betard C, Charon C, Nöthen MM, Lathrop M, Leboyer M (2006) Genome-wide scan for genes involved in bipolar affective disorder in 70 European families ascertained through a bipolar type I early-onset proband: supportive evidence for linkage at 3p14. Mol Psychiatry 11(7):685-94.

Etchegaray Jean-Pierre, Machida K. Kazuhiko, Noton Elizabeth, Constance M. Cara, Dallman Robert, Di Napoli N. Marianne, DeBruyne P. Jason, Lambert M. Christopher, Yu A. Elizabeth, Reppert M. Steven, Weaver R. David (2009) Casein Kinase 1 Delta regulates the pace of the mammalian circadian clock. Mol Cell Biol 29(14):3853-66.

Evans J, Xu K, Heron J, Enoch MA, Araya R, Lewis G, Timpson N, Davies S, Nutt D, Goldman D (2009) Emotional symptoms in children: The effect of maternal depression, life events, and COMT genotype. Am J Med Genet B Neuropsychiatr Genet 150B(2):209-18.

Evrin C, Clarke P, Zech J, Lurz R, Sun J, Uhle S, Li H, Stillman B, Speck C (2009) A double-hexameric MCM2-7 complex is loaded onto origin DNA during licensing of eukaryotic DNA replication. Proc Natl Acad Sci U S A 106(48):20240-5.

Ewald H, Degn B, Mors O, Kruse TA (1998)Support for the possible locus on chromosome 4p16 for bipolar affective disorder. Mol Psychiatry 3(5):442-8.

Ewald H, Degn B, Mors O, Kruse TA (1998) Significant linkage between bipolar affective disorder and chromosome 12q24. Psychiatr Genet. 1998 Autumn; 8(3):131-40. Abstract

Ewald H, Flint T, Kruse TA, Mors O (2002) A genome-wide scan shows significant linkage between bipolar disorder and chromosome 12q24.3 and suggestive linkage to chromosomes 1p22-21, 4p16, 6q14-22, 10q26 and 16p13.3. Mol Psychiatry 7(7):734-44.

Ewald H, Wikman FP, Teruel BM, Buttenschön HN, Torralba M, Als TD, El Daoud A, Flint TJ, Jorgensen TH, Blanco L, Kruse TA, Orntoft TF, Mors O (2005) A genome-wide search for risk genes using homozygosity mapping and microarrays with 1,494 single-nucleotide polymorphisms in 22 eastern Cuban families with bipolar disorder. Am J Med Genet B Neuropsychiatr Genet 133 B (1):25-30.

F:

Falaschi A (2000) Eukaryotic DNA replication: a model for a fixed double replisome.Trends Genet 16(2):88-92.

Fallin MD, Lasseter VK, Avramopoulos D, Nicodemus KK, Wolyniec PS, McGrath JA, Steel G, Nestadt G, Liang KY, Huganir RL, Valle D, Pulver AE (2005) Bipolar I disorder and schizophrenia: a 440-single-nucleotide polymorphism screen of 64 candidate genes among Ashkenazi Jewish case-parent trios. Am J Hum Genet 77(6):918-36.

Fan JB, Zhang CS, Gu NF, Li XW, Sun WW, Wang HY, Feng GY, St Clair D, He L (2005) Catechol-O-methyltransferase gene Val/Met functional polymorphism and risk of schizophrenia: a large-scale association study plus meta-analysis. Biol Psychiatry 57(2):139-44.

Fan Jinbo, Sklar Pamela (2008) Genetics of bipolar disorder: focus on BDNF Val66Met polymorphism. Growth factors and psychiatric disorders. Wiley, Chichester (Novartis Foundation Symposium 289) p 60-73.

Fan J, Ionita-Laza I, McQueen MB, Devlin B, Purcell S, Faraone SV, Allen MH, Bowden CL, Calabrese JR, Fossey MD, Friedman ES, Gyulai L, Hauser P, Ketter TB, Marangell LB, Miklowitz DJ, Nierenberg AA, Patel JK, Sachs GS, Thase ME, Molay FB, Escamilla MA, Nimgaonkar VL, Sklar P, Laird NM, Smoller JW (2010) Linkage disequilibrium mapping of the chromosome 6q21-22.31 bipolar I disorder susceptibility locus. Am J Med Genet B Neuropsychiatr Genet 153B(1):29-37.

Fan M, Liu B, Jiang T, Jiang X, Zhao H, Zhang J (2010) Meta-analysis of the association between the monoamine oxidase-A gene and mood disorders. Psychiatr Genet 20(1):1-7. Abstract

Fan H, Zhang F, Xu Y, Huang X, Sun G, Song Y, Long H, Liu P.An association study of DRD2 gene polymorphisms with schizophrenia in a Chinese Han population.Neurosci Lett. 2010 Jun 21;477(2):53-6. doi: 10.1016/j.neulet. 2009.11.017. Epub 2009 Nov 12.

Fathalli F, Rouleau GA, Xiong L, Tabbane K, Benkelfat C, Deguzman R, Zoltan D, Lal S, D'cruz S, Joober R (2008) No association between the DRD3 Ser9Gly polymorphism and schizophrenia. Schizophr Res 98(1-3):98-104.

Feng Y, Wigg K, King N, Vetró A, Kiss E, Kapornai K, Mayer L, Gádoros J, Kennedy JL, Kovacs M, Barr CL; International Consortium for Childhood-Onset Mood Disorders.GPR50 is not associated with childhood-onset mood disorders in a large sample of Hungarian families. Psychiatr Genet. 2007 Dec;17(6):347-50.Abstract

Fernandes BS, Gama CS, Kauer-Sant'Anna M, Lobato MI, Belmonte-de-Abreu P, Kapczinski F (2009) Serum brain-derived neurotrophic factor in bipolar and unipolar depression: a potential adjunctive tool for differential diagnosis. J Psychiatr Res 43(15):1200-4. Abstract

Ferszt R, Severus E, Bode L, Brehm M, Kühl K-P, Berzewski H, Ludwig H (1999) Activated Borna disease virus in affective disorders. Pharmacopsychiatry 32(3):93 8.

Flomen RH, Davies AF, Di Forti M, La Cascia C, Mackie-Ogilvie C, Murray R, Makoff AJ (2008) The copy number variant involving part of the alpha7 nicotinic receptor gene contains a polymorphic inversion. Eur J Hum Genet 16(11):1364-71.

Ferreira Ade A, Neves FS, da Rocha FF, Silva GS, Romano-Silva MA, Miranda DM, De Marco L, Correa H (2009) The role of 5-HTTLPR polymorphism in antidepressant-associated mania in bipolar disorder. J Affect Disord 112(1-3): 267-72.

Ferreira MA, O'Donovan MC, Meng YA, Jones IR, Ruderfer DM, Jones L, Fan J, Kirov G, Perlis RH, Green EK, Smoller JW, Grozeva D, Stone J, Nikolov I, Chambert K, Hamshere ML, Nimgaonkar VL, Moskvina V, Thase ME, Caesar S, Sachs GS, Franklin J, Gordon-Smith K, Ardlie KG, Gabriel SB, Fraser C, Blumenstiel B, Defelice M, Breen G, Gill M, Morris DW, Elkin A, Muir WJ, McGhee KA, Williamson R, MacIntyre DJ, MacLean AW, St CD, Robinson M, Van Beck M, Pereira AC, Kandaswamy R, McQuillin A, Collier DA, Bass NJ, Young AH, Lawrence J, Ferrier IN, Anjorin A, Farmer A, Curtis D, Scolnick EM, McGuffin P, Daly MJ, Corvin AP, Holmans PA, Blackwood DH, Gurling HM, Owen MJ, Purcell SM, Sklar P, Craddock N (2008) Wellcome Trust Case Control Consortium. Collaborative genome-wide association analysis supports a role for ANK3 and CACNA1C in bipolar disorder.Nat Genet 40(9):1056-8.

Fiedorowicz JG, Swartz KL (2004) The role of monoamine oxidase inhibitors in current psychiatric practice. J Psychiatr Pract 10(4):239-48.

Fountoulakis KN (2010) An update of evidence-based treatment of bipolar depression: where do we stand? Curr Opin Psychiatry 23(1):19-24.

Frazzetto G, Di Lorenzo G, Carola V, Proietti L, Sokolowska E, et al. (2007) Early Trauma and Increased Risk for Physical Aggression during Adulthood: The Moderating Role of MAOA Genotype. PLoS ONE 2(5): e486. doi:10.1371/journal.pone.0000486

Frank B, Niesler B, Nöthen MM, Neidt H, Propping P, Bondy B, Rietschel M, Maier W, Albus M, Rappold G (2004) Investigation of the human serotonin receptor gene HTR3B in bipolar affective and schizophrenic patients. Am J Med Genet B Neuropsychiatr Genet 131B(1):1-5.

Frisch A, Postilnick D, Rockah R, Michaelovsky E, Postilnick S, Birman E, Laor N, Rauchverger B, Kreinin A, Poyurovsky M, Schneidman M, Modai I, Weizman R (1999) Association of unipolar major depressive disorder with genes of the serotonergic and dopaminergic pathways. Mol Psychiatry 4(4):389-92.

Fukuo Y, Kishi T, Yoshimura R, Kitajima T, Okochi T, Yamanouchi Y, Kinoshita Y, Kawashima K, Naitoh H, Umene-Nakano W, Inada T, Kunugi H, Kato T, Yoshikawa T, Ujike H, Nakamura J, Ozaki N, Iwata N.Serotonin 6 receptor gene and mood disorders: case-control study and meta-analysis. Neurosci Res. 2010 Jul;67(3):250-5. doi: 10.1016/j.neures.2010.04.003. Epub 2010 Apr 13.

Furlong RA, Ho L, Rubinsztein JS, Walsh C, Paykel ES, Rubinsztein DC (1998) No association of the tryptophan hydroxylase gene with bipolar affective disorder, unipolar affective disorder, or suicidal behaviour in major affective disorder.Am J Med Genet 81(3):245-7.

Furlong RA, Ho L, Rubinsztein JS, Walsh C, Paykel ES, Rubinsztein DC (1999) Analysis of the Monoamine Oxidase A (MAOA) Gene in Bipolar Affective Disorder by Association Studies, Meta-Analyses, and Sequencing of the Promoter. American Journal of Medical Genetics (Neuropsychiatric Genetics) 88:398–406

Furlong RA, Ho L, Walsh C, Rubinsztein JS, Jain S, Paykel ES, Easton DF, Rubinsztein DC (1998) Analysis and meta-analysis of two serotonin transporter gene polymorphisms in bipolar and unipolar affective disorders. Am J Med Genet 81(1):58-63.

Furlong RA, Coleman TA, Ho L, Rubinsztein JS, Walsh C, Paykel ES, Rubinsztein DC (1998) No association of a functional polymorphism in the dopamine D2 receptor promoter region with bipolar or unipolar affective disorders. Am J Med Genet 81(5):385-7.

G:

Galfalvy H, Huang YY, Oquendo MA, Currier D, Mann JJ (2009) Increased risk of suicide attempt in mood disorders and TPH1 genotype. J Affect Disord 115(3):331-8.

Garner C, McInnes LA, Service SK, Spesny M, Fournier E, Leon P, Freimer NB (2001) Linkage analysis of a complex pedigree with severe bipolar disorder, using a Markov chain Monte Carlo method. Am J Hum Genet 68(4):1061-4.

Gaysina D, Cohen-Woods S, Chow PC, Martucci L, Schosser A, Ball HA, Tozzi F, Perry J, Muglia P, Craig IW, McGuffin P, Farmer A (2009) Association of the dystrobrevin binding protein 1 gene (DTNBP1) in a bipolar case-control study (BACCS). Am J Med Genet B Neuropsychiatr Genet 150B (6):836-44.

Geller B, Cook EH Jr (1999) Serotonin transporter gene (HTTLPR) is not in linkage disequilibrium with prepubertal and early adolescent bipolarity. Biol Psychiatry 45(9):1230-3.

Geller B, Badner JA, Tillman R, Christian SL, Bolhofner K, Cook EH Jr (2004) Linkage Disequilibrium of the Brain-derived neurotrophic factor Val66Met polymorphism in children with a prepubertal and early adolescent bipolar disorder phenotype. Am J Psychiatry 161(9):1698-700.

Genome wide association study of 14,000 cases of seven common diseases and 3,000 shared controls (2007) Wellcome Trust Case Control Consortium. Nature 447(7145):661-78

Gekakis N, Staknis D, Nguyen HB, Davis FC, Wilsbacher LD, King DP, Takahashi JS, Weitz CJ (1998) Role of the CLOCK protein in the mammalian circadian mechanism. Science 280(5369):1564-9.

Geller B, Cook EH Jr (2000) Ultradian rapid cycling in prepubertal and early adolescent bipolarity is not in transmission disequilibrium with val/met COMT alleles. Biol Psychiatry 47(7):605-9.

Georgieva L, Dimitrova A, Nikolov I, Koleva S, Tsvetkova R, Owen MJ, Toncheva D, Kirov G (2002) Dopamine transporter gene (DAT1) VNTR polymorphism in major psychiatric disorders: family-based association study in the Bulgarian population. Acta Psychiatr Scand 105(5):396-9.

Georgieva L, Dimitrova A, Ivanov D, Nikolov I, Williams NM, Grozeva D, Zaharieva I, Toncheva D, Owen MJ, Kirov G, O'Donovan MC (2008) Support for neuregulin 1 as a susceptibility gene for bipolar disorder and schizophrenia. Biol Psychiatry 64(5):419-27.

Georgi A, Jamra RA, Schumacher J, Becker T, Schmael C, Deschner M, Höfels S, Wulff M, Schwarz M, Klopp N, Illig T, Propping P, Cichon S, Nöthen MM, Rietschel M, Schulze TG.No association between genetic variants at the GRIN1 gene and bipolar disorder in a German sample. Psychiatr Genet. 2006 Oct;16(5):183-4.

Ghadirivasfi M, Nohesara S, Ahmadkhaniha HR, Eskandari MR, Mostafavi S, Thiagalingam S, Abdolmaleky HM.Hypomethylation of the serotonin receptor type-2A Gene (HTR2A) at T102C polymorphic site in DNA derived from the saliva of patients with schizophrenia and bipolar disorder. Am J Med Genet

B Neuropsychiatr Genet. 2011 Jul;156B(5):536-45. doi: 10.1002/ajmg.b. 31192. Epub 2011 May 19.
Gillanders EM, Masiello A, Gildea D, Umayam L, Duggal P, Jones MP, Klein AP, Freas-Lutz D, Ibay G, Trout K, Wolfsberg TG, Trent JM, Bailey-Wilson JE, Baxevanis AD (2004) GeneLink: a database to facilitate genetic studies of complex traits. BMC Genomics 5(1):81.
Gillespie CF, Phifer J, Bradley B, Ressler KJ (2009) Risk and resilience: genetic and environmental influences on development of the stress response. Depress Anxiety 26(11):984-92.
Girault JA, Greengard P.The neurobiology of dopamine signaling. Arch Neurol. 2004 May;61(5):641-4.
Gizatullin R, Zaboli G, Jönsson EG, Asberg M, Leopardi R (2006) Haplotype analysis reveals tryptophan hydroxylase (TPH) 1 gene variants associated with major depression. Biol Psychiatry 59(4):295-300.
Glaser B, Kirov G, Green E, Craddock N, Owen MJ (2005) Linkage disequilibrium mapping of bipolar affective disorder at 12q23-q24 provides evidence for association at CUX2 and FLJ32356. Am J Med Genet B Neuropsychiatr Genet 132B(1):38-45.
Glatt SJ, Faraone SV, Tsuang MT (2003) CAG-repeat length in exon 1 of KCNN3 does not influence risk for schizophrenia or bipolar disorder: a meta-analysis of association studies. Am J Med Genet B Neuropsychiatr Genet 121B(1):14-20.
Glazier AM, Nadeau JH, Aitman TJ (2002) Finding genes that underlie complex traits. Science 298(5602):2345-9.
Goldberg TE, Kotov R, Lee AT, Gregersen PK, Lencz T, Bromet E, Malhotra AK (2009) The serotonin transporter gene and disease modification in psychosis: evidence for systematic differences in allelic directionality at the 5-HTTLPR locus. Schizophr Res 111(1-3):103-8.
Goes FS, Sanders LL, Potash JB (2008) The genetics of psychotic bipolar disorder. Curr Psychiatry Rep 10(2):178-89.
Goes FS, Willour VL, Zandi PP, Belmonte PL, MacKinnon DF, Mondimore FM, Schweizer B, Gershon ES, McMahon FJ, Potash JB (2009) Bipolar Disorder Phenome Group; NIMH Genetics Initiative Bipolar Disorder Consortium.Family-based association study of Neuregulin 1 with psychotic bipolar disorder. Am J Med Genet B Neuropsychiatr Genet 150B(5):693-702.
Goes FS, Hamshere ML, Seifuddin F, Pirooznia M, Belmonte-Mahon P, Breuer R, Schulze T, Nöthen M, Cichon S, Rietschel M, Holmans P, Zandi PP; Bipolar Genome Study (BiGS), Craddock N, Potash JB.Genome-wide association of mood-incongruent psychotic bipolar disorder. Transl Psychiatry. 2012 Oct 23;2:e180. doi: 10.1038/tp.2012.106.

Gomez L, Wigg K, Feng Y, Kiss E, Kapornai K, Tamás Z, Mayer L, Baji I, Daróczi G, Benák I, Kothencné VO, Dombovári E, Kaczvinszk E, Besnyo M, Gádoros J, King N, Székely J, Kovacs M, Vetró A, Kennedy JL, Barr CL (2009) G72/G30 (DAOA) and juvenile-onset mood disorders. Am J Med Genet B Neuropsychiatr Genet 150B(7):1007-12.

Gonçalves VF, Tiwari AK, de Luca V, Kong SL, Zai C, Tampakeras M, Mackenzie B, Sun L, Kennedy JL.DRD4 VNTR polymorphism and age at onset of severe mental illnesses. Neurosci Lett. 2012 Jun 21;519(1):9-13. doi: 10.1016/j.neulet.2012.04.027. Epub 2012 Apr 20.

Göthert M, Propping P, Bönisch H, Brüss M, Nöthen MM (1998) Genetic variation in human 5-HT receptors: potential pathogenetic and pharmacological role. Ann N Y Acad Sci 861:26-30.

Goghari VM, Sponheim SR (2008) Differential association of the COMT Val158Met polymorphism with clinical phenotypes in schizophrenia and bipolar disorder. Schizophr Res 103(1-3):186-91.

Gratacòs M, Costas J, de Cid R, Bayés M, González JR, Baca-García E, de Diego Y, Fernández-Aranda F, Fernández-Piqueras J, Guitart M, Martín-Santos R, Martorell L, Menchón JM, Roca M, Sáiz-Ruiz J, Sanjuán J, Torrens M, Urretavizcaya M, Valero J, Vilella E, Estivill X, Carracedo A (2009) Psychiatric Genetics Network Group.Identification of new putative susceptibility genes for several psychiatric disorders by association analysis of regulatory and non-synonymous SNPs of 306 genes involved in neurotransmission and neurodevelopment. Am J Med Genet B Neuropsychiatr Genet 150B(6):808-16.

Green MR (2000) TBP-associated factors (TAFIIs): multiple, selective transcriptional mediators in common complexes. Trends Biochem Sci 25(2):59-63.

Green EK, Raybould R, Macgregor S, Hyde S, Young AH, O'Donovan MC, Owen MJ, Kirov G, Jones L, Jones I, Craddock N (2006) Genetic variation of brain-derived neurotrophic factor (BDNF) in bipolar disorder. Case control study of over 3000 individuals from the UK.. British journal of Psychiatry 188:21-25

Green E, Elvidge G, Jacobsen N, Glaser B, Jones I, O'Donovan MC, Kirov G, Owen MJ, Craddock N (2005) Localization of bipolar susceptibility locus by molecular genetic analysis of the chromosome 12q23-q24 region in two pedigrees with bipolar disorder and Darier's disease. Am J Psychiatry 162(1):35-42.

Green EK, Raybould R, Macgregor S, Gordon-Smith K, Heron J, Hyde S, Grozeva D, Hamshere M, Williams N, Owen MJ, O'Donovan MC, Jones L, Jones I, Kirov G, Craddock N (2005) Operation of the schizophrenia susceptibility gene, neuregulin 1, across traditional diagnostic boundaries to increase risk for bipolar disorder. Arch Gen Psychiatry 62(6):642-8.

Green EK, Grozeva D, Raybould R, Elvidge G, Macgregor S, Craig I, Farmer A, McGuffin P, Forty L, Jones L, Jones I, O'Donovan MC, Owen MJ, Kirov G, Craddock N (2009) P2RX7: A bipolar and unipolar disorder candidate susceptibility gene? Am J Med Genet B Neuropsychiatr Genet150B(8):1063-9.

Green EK, Grozeva D, Jones I, Jones L, Kirov G, Caesar S, Gordon-Smith K, Fraser C, Forty L, Russell E, Hamshere ML, Moskvina V, Nikolov I, Farmer A, McGuffin P; Wellcome Trust Case Control Consortium5, Holmans PA, Owen MJ, O'Donovan MC, Craddock N (2009) The bipolar disorder risk allele at CACNA1C also confers risk of recurrent major depression and of schizophrenia. Mol Psychiatry.

Green EK, Grozeva D, Moskvina V, Hamshere ML, Jones IR, Jones L, Forty L, Caesar S, Gordon-Smith K, Fraser C, Russell E, St Clair D, Young AH, Ferrier N, Farmer A, McGuffin P, Holmans PA, Owen MJ, O'Donovan MC, Craddock N. Variation at the GABAA receptor gene, Rho 1 (GABRR1) associated with susceptibility to bipolar schizoaffective disorder. Am J Med Genet B Neuropsychiatr Genet. 2010 Oct 5;153B(7):1347-9. doi: 10.1002/ajmg.b.31108.

Green EK, Hamshere M, Forty L, Gordon-Smith K, Fraser C, Russell E, Grozeva D, Kirov G, Holmans P, Moran JL, Purcell S, Sklar P, Owen MJ, O'Donovan MC, Jones L; WTCCC, Jones IR, Craddock N. Replication of bipolar disorder susceptibility alleles and identification of two novel genome-wide significant associations in a new bipolar disorder case-control sample. Mol Psychiatry. 2012 Oct 16. doi: 10.1038/mp.2012.142. [Epub ahead of print]

Greenwood, TA, Akiskal, HS, Akiskal, KK, Bipolar Genome Study, Kelsoe, JR, 2012. Genome-Wide Association Study of Temperament in Bipolar Disorder Reveals Significant Associations with Three Novel Loci. Biol. Psychiatry.

Greenwood TA, Joo EJ, Shekhtman T, Sadovnick AD, Remick RA, Keck PE, McElroy SL, Kelsoe JR.Association of dopamine transporter gene variants with childhood ADHD features in bipolar disorder. Am J Med Genet B Neuropsychiatr Genet. 2012 Dec 19. doi: 10.1002/ajmg.b.32108.

Griffiths AJF, Miller JH, Suzuki DT, Lewontin RC, Gelbart WM (1993). "Chapter 5". An Introduction to Genetic Analysis (5th ed.). New York: WH Freeman and Company. ISBN 0-7167-2285-2.

Griffiths, A. J. F.; Miller, J. H.; Suzuki, D. T.; Lewontin, R. C.; Gelbart, W. M. Derivation of mapping function, from Introduction to Genetic Analysis. New York: W. H. Freeman & Co.; 1999

Grigoroiu-Serbanescu M, Herms S, Diaconu CC, Jamra RA, Meier S, Bleotu C, Neagu AI, Prelipceanu D, Sima D, Gherghel M, Mihailescu R, Rietschel M, Nöthen MM, Cichon S, Mühleisen TW. Possible association of different

G72/G30 SNPs with mood episodes and persecutory delusions in bipolar I Romanian patients.Prog Neuropsychopharmacol Biol Psychiatry. 2010 May 30;34(4):657-63. doi: 10.1016/j.pnpbp.2010.03.008. Epub 2010 Mar 15.
Grigoroiu-Serbanescu M, Herms S, Mühleisen TW, Georgi A, Diaconu CC, Strohmaier J, Czerski P, Hauser J, Leszczynska-Rodziewicz A, Jamra RA, Babadjanova G, Tiganov A, Krasnov V, Kapiletti S, Neagu AI, Vollmer J, Breuer R, Rietschel M, Nöthen MM, Cichon S, Propping P, Nöthen MM, Cichon S (2009) Variation in P2RX7 candidate gene (rs2230912) is not associated with bipolar I disorder and unipolar major depression in four European samples. Am J Med Genet B Neuropsychiatr Genet 150B(7):1017-21
Grigoroiu-Serbanescu M, Diaconu CC, Herms S, Bleotu C, Vollmer J, Mühleisen TW, Prelipceanu D, Priebe L, Mihailescu R, Georgescu MJ, Sima D, Grimberg M, Nöthen MM, Cichon S.Investigation of the tryptophan hydroxylase 2 gene in bipolar I disorder in the Romanian population. Psychiatr Genet. 2008 Oct;18(5):240-7. doi: 10.1097/YPG.0b013e3283053045
Grünhage F, Schulze TG, Müller DJ, Lanczik M, Franzek E, Albus M, Borrmann-Hassenbach M, Knapp M, Cichon S, Maier W, Rietschel M, Propping P, Nöthen MM (2000) Systematic screening for DNA sequence variation in the coding region of the human dopamine transporter gene (DAT1). Mol Psychiatry 5(3):275-82.
Grzywacz A, Samochowiec A, Ciechanowicz A, Samochowiec J.Family-based study of brain-derived neurotrophic factor (BDNF) gene polymorphism in alcohol dependence. Pharmacol Rep. 2010 Sep-Oct;62(5):938-41.
Gu Y, Yun L, Tian Y, Hu Z (2009) Association between COMT gene and Chinese male schizophrenic patients with violent behavior. Med Sci Monit15(9): CR484-9.
Gurling HM, Kalsi G, Brynjolfson J, Sigmundsson T, Sherrington R, Mankoo BS, Read T, Murphy P, Blaveri E, McQuillin A, Petursson H, Curtis D (2001) Genomewide genetic linkage analysis confirms the presence of susceptibility loci for schizophrenia, on chromosomes 1q32.2, 5q33.2, and 8p21-22 and provides support for linkage to schizophrenia, on chromosomes 11q23.3-24 and 20q12.1-11.23.Am J Hum Genet 68(3):661-73.
Gutiérrez B, Bertranpetit J, Guillamat R, Vallès V, Arranz MJ, Kerwin R, Fañanás L (1997) Association analysis of the catechol O-methyltransferase gene and bipolar affective disorder. Am J Psychiatry 154(1):113-5.
Gutiérrez B, Bertranpetit J, Collier D, Arranz MJ, Vallès V, Guillamat R, Van Os J, Fañanás L (1997) Genetic variation of the 5-HT2A receptor gene and bipolar affective disorder. Hum Genet 100(5-6):582-4.

Gutiérrez B, Pintor L, Gastó C, Rosa A, Bertranpetit J, Vieta E, Fañanás L (1998) Variability in the serotonin transporter gene and increased risk for major depression with melancholia. Hum Genet 103(3):319-22.

Gutiérrez B, Arias B, Papiol S, Rosa A, Fañanás L (2001) Association study between novel promoter variants at the 5-HT2C receptor gene and human patients with bipolar affective disorder. Neurosci Lett 309(2):135-7.

H:

Hadley D, Hoff M, Holik J, Reimherr F, Wender P, Coon H, Byerley W (1995) Manic-depression and the norepinephrine transporter gene. Hum Hered 45(3):165-8. Abstract

Haenisch B, Linsel K, Brüss M, Gilsbach R, Propping P, Nöthen MM, Rietschel M, Fimmers R, Maier W, Zobel A, Höfels S, Guttenthaler V, Göthert M, Bönisch H (2009) Association of major depression with rare functional variants in norepinephrine transporter and serotonin1A receptor genes.Am J Med Genet B Neuropsychiatr Genet 150B(7):1013-6.

Haque FN, Gottesman II, Wong AH (2009) Not really identical: epigenetic differences in monozygotic twins and implications for twin studies in psychiatry. Am J Med Genet C Semin Med Genet 151C(2):136-41.

Hamilton SP (2008) Schizophrenia Candidate Genes: Are We Really Coming Up Blank? Am J Psychiatry 165:4

Hammer C, Cichon S, Mühleisen TW, Haenisch B, Degenhardt F, Mattheisen M, Breuer R, Witt SH, Strohmaier J, Oruc L, Rivas F, Babadjanova G, Grigoroiu-Serbanescu M, Hauser J, Röth R, Rappold G, Rietschel M, Nöthen MM, Niesler B. Replication of functional serotonin receptor type 3A and B variants in bipolar affective disorder: a European multicenter study.Transl Psychiatry. 2012 Apr 17;2:e103. doi: 10.1038/tp.2012.30.

Hampp G, Albrecht U (2008) The circadian clock and mood-related behavior. Commun Integr Biol 1(1):1-3.

Hampp G, Ripperger JA, Houben T, Schmutz I, Blex C, Perreau-Lenz S, Brunk I, Spanagel R, Ahnert-Hilger G, Meijer JH, Albrecht U (2008) Regulation of Monoamine Oxidase A by Circadian-Clock Components Implies Clock Influence on Mood. Current Biology 18:678–683

Hamshere ML, Bennett P, Williams N, Segurado R, Cardno A, Norton N, Lambert D, Williams H, Kirov G, Corvin A, Holmans P, Jones L, Jones I, Gill M, O'Donovan MC, Owen MJ, Craddock N (2005) Genomewide linkage scan in schizoaffective disorder: significant evidence for linkage at 1q42 close to DISC1, and suggestive evidence at 22q11 and 19p13.Arch Gen Psychiatry 62(10):1081 8

Hamshere ML, Walters JT, Smith R, Richards AL, Green E, Grozeva D, Jones I, Forty L, Jones L, Gordon-Smith K, Riley B, O'Neill T, Kendler KS, Sklar P, Purcell S, Kranz J; The Schizophrenia Psychiatric Genome-wide Association Study Consortium (PGC), Wellcome Trust Case Control Consortium+ (WTCCC+), Wellcome Trust Case Control Consortium 2 (WTCCC2), Morris D, Gill M, Holmans P, Craddock N, Corvin A, Owen MJ, O'Donovan MCGenome-wide significant associations in schizophrenia to ITIH3/4, CACNA1C and SDCCAG8, and extensive replication of associations reported by the Schizophrenia PGC. Mol Psychiatry. 2012 May 22. doi: 10.1038/mp.2012.67.

Harvey M, Shink E, Tremblay M, Gagné B, Raymond C, Labbé M, Walther DJ, Bader M, Barden N.Support for the involvement of TPH2 gene in affective disorders. Mol Psychiatry. 2004 Nov;9(11):980-1.

Harvey M, Gagné B, Labbé M, Barden N. Polymorphisms in the neuronal isoform of tryptophan hydroxylase 2 are associated with bipolar disorder in French Canadian pedigrees.Psychiatr Genet. 2007 Feb;17(1):17-22.

Hashimoto K, Shimizu E, Iyo M (2004) Critical role of brain-derived neurotrophic factor in mood disorders. Brain research Reviews 45:104-114.

Hashimoto R, Okada T, Kato T, Kosuga A, Tatsumi M, Kamijima K, Kunugi H (2005) The breakpoint cluster region gene on chromosome 22q11 is associated with bipolar disorder. Biol Psychiatry 57(10):1097-102.

Hashimoto R, Numakawa T, Ohnishi T, Kumamaru E, Yagasaki Y, Ishimoto T, Mori T, Nemoto K, Adachi N, Izumi A, Chiba S, Noguchi H, Suzuki T, Iwata N, Ozaki N, Taguchi T, Kamiya A, Kosuga A, Tatsumi M, Kamijima K, Weinberger DR, Sawa A, Kunugi H (2006) Impact of the DISC1 Ser704Cys polymorphism on risk for major depression, brain morphology and ERK signaling. Hum Mol Genet 15(20):3024-33.

Haustgen T, Akiskal H (2006) French antecedents of "contemporary" concepts in the American Psychiatric Association's classification of bipolar (mood) disorders. J Affect Disord 96(3):149-63.

Heiden A, Schüssler P, Itzlinger U, Leisch F, Scharfetter J, Gebhardt C, Fuchs K, Willeit M, Nilsson L, Miller-Reiter E, Stompe T, Meszaros K, Sieghart W, Hornik K, Kasper S, Aschauer HN (2000)Association studies of candidate genes in bipolar disorders. Neuropsychobiology42:18-21.

Heils A, Teufel A, Petri S, Stöber G, Riederer P, Bengel D, Lesch KP (1996) Allelic variation of human serotonin transporter gene expression. J Neurochem 66(6):2621-4.

Hejjas K, Szekely A, Domotor E, Halmai Z, Balogh G, Schilling B, Sarosi A, Faludi G, Sasvari-Szekely M, Nemoda Z (2009) Association between depression and the Gln460Arg polymorphism of P2RX7 gene: a dimensional approach. Am J Med Genet B Neuropsychiatr Genet 150B(2):295-9.

Hamshere ML, Bennett P, Williams N, Segurado R, Cardno A, Norton N, Lambert D, Williams H, Kirov G, Corvin A, Holmans P, Jones L, Jones I, Gill M, O'Donovan MC, Owen MJ, Craddock N (2005) Genomewide linkage scan in schizoaffective disorder: significant evidence for linkage at 1q42 close to DISC1, and suggestive evidence at 22q11 and 19p13.Arch Gen Psychiatry 62(10):1081-8.

Hennah W, Porteous D (2009)The DISC1 pathway modulates expression of neurodevelopmental, synaptogenic and sensory perception genes. PLoS One 4(3):e4906.

Herzberg I, Jasinska A, García J, Jawaheer D, Service S, Kremeyer B, Duque C, Parra MV, Vega J, Ortiz D, Carvajal L, Polanco G, Restrepo GJ, López C, Palacio C, Levinson M, Aldana I, Mathews C, Davanzo P, Molina J, Fournier E, Bejarano J, Ramírez M, Ortiz CA, Araya X, Sabatti C, Reus V, Macaya G, Bedoya G, Ospina J, Freimer N, Ruiz-Linares A (2006) Convergent linkage evidence from two Latin-American population isolates supports the presence of a susceptibility locus for bipolar disorder in 5q31-34.Hum Mol Genet 15(21):3146-53.

Hettema JM, An SS, van den Oord EJ, Neale MC, Kendler KS, Chen X (2008) Association study between the serotonin 1A receptor (HTR1A) gene and neuroticism, major depression, and anxiety disorders. Am J Med Genet B Neuropsychiatr Genet 147B(5):661-6.

Hilt LM, Sander LC, Nolen-Hoeksema S, Simen AA (2007) The BDNF Val66Met polymorphism predicts rumination and depression differently in young adolescent girls and their mothers. Neurosci Lett 429(1):12-6.

Hinds HL, Hendriks RW, Craig IW, Chen ZY (1992) Characterization of a highly polymorphic region near the first exon of the human MAOA gene containing a GT dinucleotide and a novel VNTR motif. Genomics 13(3):896-7.

Hippius H, Müller N (2008) The work of Emil Kraepelin and his research group in München. Eur Arch Psychiatry Clin Neurosci 258 (2):3-11.

Hoehe MR, Wendel B, Grunewald I, Chiaroni P, Levy N, Morris-Rosendahl D, Macher JP, Sander T, Crocq MA (1998) Serotonin transporter (5-HTT) gene polymorphisms are not associated with susceptibility to mood disorders. Am J Med Genet 81(1):1-3.

Holmes A (2009) Genetic variation in cortico-amygdala serotonin function and risk for stress-related disease. Neurosci Biobehav Rev. Author manuscript; available in PMC 2009 September 1.

Hong CJ, Tsai SJ, Cheng CY, Liao WY, Song HL, Lai HC (1999) Association analysis of the 5-HT(6) receptor polymorphism (C267T) in mood disorders. Am J Med Genet 88(6):601-2.

Hong CJ, Huo SJ, Yen FC, Tung CL, Pan GM, Tsai SJ (2003) Association Study of a Brain-Derived Neurotrophic Factor Genetic Polymorphism and Mood Disorders, Age of Onset and Suicidal Behavior. Neuropsychobiology 48:186-189

Hong KS, McInnes LA, Service SK, Song T, Lucas J, Silva S, Fournier E, León P, Molina J, Reus VI, Sandkuijl LA, Freimer NB (2004) Genetic mapping using haplotype and model-free linkage analysis supports previous evidence for a locus predisposing to severe bipolar disorder at 5q31-33. Am J Med Genet B Neuropsychiatr Genet 125B(1):83-6.

Hodgkinson CA, Goldman D, Jaeger J, Persaud S, Kane JM, Lipsky RH, Malhotra AK (2004) Disrupted in schizophrenia 1 (DISC1): association with schizophrenia, schizoaffective disorder, and bipolar disorder. Am J Hum Genet 75(5):862-72.

Hoenicka J, Garrido E, Martínez I, Ponce G, Aragüés M, Rodríguez-Jiménez R, España-Serrano L, Alvira-Botero X, Santos JL, Rubio G, Jiménez-Arriero MA, Palomo T; PARGPARG (2010) Gender-specific COMT Val158Met polymorphism association in Spanish schizophrenic patients.Am J Med Genet B Neuropsychiatr Genet153B(1):79-85.

Horsthemke B, Wagstaff J (2008) Mechanisms of imprinting of the Prader-Willi/Angelman region. Am J Med Genet A 146A(16):2041-52.

Hotamisligil GS, Breakefield XO (1991) Human monoamine oxidase A gene determines levels of enzyme activity. Am J Hum Genet 49:383–392.

Hu MC, Lee SY, Wang TY, Chen SL, Chang YH, Chen SH, Chu CH, Wang CL, Lee IH, Yeh TL, Yang YK, Lu RB.Association study of DRD2 and MAOA genes with subtyped alcoholism comorbid with bipolar disorder in Han Chinese. Prog Neuropsychopharmacol Biol Psychiatry. 2013 Jan 10;40:144-8. doi: 10.1016/j.pnpbp.2012.09.014. Epub 2012 Oct 5.

Huang YY, Oquendo MA, Friedman JM, Greenhill LL, Brodsky B, Malone KM, Khait V, Mann JJ (2003) Substance abuse disorder and major depression are associated with the human 5-HT1B receptor gene (HTR1B) G861C polymorphism. Neuropsychopharmacology 28(1):163-9.

Huang SY, Lin MT, Shy MJ, Lin WW, Lin FY, Lu RB (2008) Neither single-marker nor haplotype analyses support an association between monoamine oxidase A gene and bipolar disorder. Eur Arch Psychiatry Clin Neurosci 258:350–356

Hyong Jin Cho, Helen Lavretsky, Richard Olmstead, Myron J. Levin, Michael N. Oxman, and Michael R. Irwin (2008) Sleep Disturbance and Depression Recurrence in Community-Dwelling Older Adults: A Prospective Study. Am J Psychiatry 165(12): 1543–1550.

I:

Ikeda M, Iwata N, Suzuki T, Kitajima T, Yamanouchi Y, Kinoshita Y, Ozaki N (2006) No association of serotonin transporter gene (SLC6A4) with schizophrenia and bipolar disorder in Japanese patients: association analysis based on linkage disequilibrium. J Neural Transm 113(7):899-905.

Illi A, Setälä-Soikkeli E, Viikki M, Poutanen O, Huhtala H, Mononen N, Lehtimäki T, Leinonen E, Kampman O (2009) 5-HTR1A, 5-HTR2A, 5-HTR6, TPH1 and TPH2 polymorphisms and major depression. Neuroreport 20(12):1125-8.

Ivanova MA, Christova TN, Asan TS, Djurova NA, Alexiev SS, Kostov CS, Chorbov VM, Stoyanova VS, Onchev GN, Kancheva DM, Krastev SK, Vladimirova RK, Kremensky IM, Mitev V, Milanova VK, Kaneva RP. Evidence of an association between **bipolar disorder** and rs16917237 in the **BDNF** gene in a Bulgarian sample.Psychiatr Genet. 2012 Dec 30

J:

Jablensky A (1999) The conflict of the nosologists: views on schizophrenia and manic-depressive illness in the early part of the 20th century. Schizophr Res 39(2):95-100.

Jacobsen NJ, Franks EK, Elvidge G, Jones I, McCandless F, O'Donovan MC, Owen MJ, Craddock N (2001) Exclusion of the Darier's disease gene, ATP2A2, as a common susceptibility gene for bipolar disorder. Mol Psychiatry 6(1):92-7.

Jacobsen NJ, Elvidge G, Franks EK, O'Donovan MC, Craddock N, Owen MJ (2001) CUX2, a potential regulator of NCAM expression: genomic characterization and analysis as a positional candidate susceptibility gene for bi-polar disorder. Am J Med Genet 105(3):295-300.

Jin DK, Hwang HZ, Oh MR, Kim JS, Lee M, Kim S, Lim SW, Seo MY, Kim JH, Kim DK (2001) CAG repeats of CTG18.1 and KCNN3 in Korean patients with bipolar affective disorder. J Affect Disord 66(1):19-24.

Jivotovskaya AV, Valásek L, Hinnebusch AG, Nielsen KH (2006) Eukaryotic translation initiation factor 3 (eIF3) and eIF2 can promote mRNA binding to 40S subunits independently of eIF4G in yeast. Mol Cell Biol 26(4):1355-72.

Jönsson EG, Norton N, Forslund K, Mattila-Evenden M, Rylander G, Asberg M, Owen MJ, Sedvall GC (2003) Association between a promoter variant in the monoamine oxidase A gene and schizophrenia. Schizophr Res 61(1):31-7.

Jönsson EG, Larsson K, Vares M, Hansen T, Wang AG, Djurovic S, Rønningen KS, Andreassen OA, Agartz I, Werge T, Terenius L, Hall H (2008) Two methylenetetrahydrofolate reductase gene (MTHFR) polymorphisms, schizophrenia and bipolar disorder: an association study. Am J Med Genet B Neuropsychiatr Genet 147B(6):976-82.

Jönsson EG, Saetre P, Vares M, Andreou D, Larsson K, Timm S, Rasmussen HB, Djurovic S, Melle I, Andreassen OA, Agartz I, Werge T, Hall H, Terenius L (2009) DTNBP1, NRG1, DAOA, DAO and GRM3 polymorphisms and schizophrenia: an association study. Neuropsychobiology 59(3):142-50.

Joo EJ, Lee KY, Jeong SH, Chang JS, Ahn YM, Koo YJ, Kim YS (2007) Dysbindin gene variants are associated with bipolar I disorder in a Korean population. Neurosci Lett 418(3):272-5.

Johansson C, Willeit M, Smedh C, Ekholm J, Paunio T, Kieseppä T, Lichtermann D, Praschak-Rieder N, Neumeister A, Nilsson LG, Kasper S, Peltonen L, Adolfsson R, Schalling M, Partonen T (2003) Circadian clock-related polymorphisms in seasonal affective disorder and their relevance to diurnal preference. Neuropsychopharmacology 28(4):734-9.

Jokela M, Lehtimäki T, Keltikangas-Järvinen L (2007) The influence of urban/rural residency on depressive symptoms is moderated by the serotonin receptor 2A gene. Am J Med Genet B Neuropsychiatr Genet 144B(7):918-22.

Jones I, Jacobsen N, Green EK, Elvidge GP, Owen MJ, Craddock N (2002) Evidence for familial cosegregation of major affective disorder and genetic markers flanking the gene for Darier's disease. Mol Psychiatry 7(4):424-7.

Juven-Gershon T, Hsu JY, Theisen JW, Kadonaga JT (2008) The RNA polymerase II core promoter – the gateway to transcription.Curr Opin Cell Biol 20(3):253-9.

K:

Kadonaga JT (2002) The DPE, a core promoter element for transcription by RNA polymerase II. Exp Mol Med 34(4):259-64.

Kealey C, Roche S, Claffey E, McKeon P. Linkage and candidate gene analysis of 14q22-24 in bipolar disorder: support for GCHI as a novel susceptibility gene. Am J Med Genet B Neuropsychiatr Genet. 2005 Jul 5;136B(1):75-80.

Kapoor S (2009) Systemic and Psychiatric Disorders Associated With Polymorphisms of the P2RX7 Gene. Am J Med Genet Part B 150B:597-598.

Kamiya A, Tomoda T, Chang J, Takaki M, Zhan C, Morita M, Cascio MB, Elashvili S, Koizumi H, Takanezawa Y, Dickerson F, Yolken R, Arai H, Sawa A (2006) DISC1-NDEL1/NUDEL protein interaction, an essential component for neurite outgrowth, is modulated by genetic variations of DISC1. Hum Mol Genet 15(22):3313-23.

Kan R, Wang B, Zhang C, Yang Z, Ji S, Lu Z, Zheng C, Jin F, Wang L (2004) Association of the HTR6 polymorphism C267T with late-onset Alzheimer's disease in Chinese. Neurosci Lett 372(1-2):27-9.

Kanazawa, Tetsufumi, Glatt, Stephen, Kia-Keating, Brett, Yoneda, Hiroshi, Tsuang, Ming (2007) Meta-analysis reveals no association of the Val66Met polymorphism of brain-derived neurotrophic factor with either schizophrenia or bipolar disorder. Psychiatric Genetics. 17(3):165-170.

Kaneko K, Yamada T, Tsukita S, Takahashi K, Ishigaki Y, Oka Y, Katagiri H (2009) Obesity alters circadian expressions of molecular clock genes in the brainstem. Brain Res 1263:58-68.

Kapfhammer HP, Möller HJ, Laux G (2008) Psychiatrie und Psychotherapie. 3.Auflage. Springer Verlag.

Kato T, Iwayama Y, Kakiuchi C, Iwamoto K, Yamada K, Minabe Y, Nakamura K, Mori N, Fujii K, Nanko S, Yoshikawa T (2005) Gene expression and association analyses of LIM (PDLIM5) in bipolar disorder and schizophrenia. Mol Psychiatry 10(11):1045-55.Abstract

Kato M, Fukuda T, Wakeno M, Okugawa G, Takekita Y, Watanabe S, Yamashita M, Hosoi Y, Azuma J, Kinoshita T, Serretti A (2009) Effect of 5-HT1A Gene Polymorphisms on Antidepressant Response in Major DepressiveDisorder. Am J Med Genet Part B 150B:115–123.

Kawada Y, Hattori M, Dai XY, Nanko S (1995) Possible association between monoamine oxidase A gene and bipolar affective disorder. Am J Hum Genet 56(1):335-6.

Kawashima K, Ikeda M, Kishi T, Kitajima T, Yamanouchi Y, Kinoshita Y, Okochi T, Aleksic B, Tomita M, Okada T, Kunugi H, Inada T, Ozaki N, Iwata N (2009) BDNF is not associated with schizophrenia: data from a Japanese population study and meta-analysis. Schizophr Res. 2009 Jul;112(1-3):72-9.

Kishi T, Yoshimura R, Kitajima T, Okochi T, Okumura T, Tsunoka T, Yamanouchi Y, Kinoshita Y, Kawashima K, Naitoh H, Nakamura J, Ozaki N, Iwata N. HTR2A is associated with SSRI response in major depressive disorder in a Japanese cohort.Neuromolecular Med. 2010 Sep;12(3):237-42. doi: 10.1007/s12017-009-8105-y. Epub 2009 Nov 24.

Kauer-Sant'Anna M, Kapczinski F, Andreazza AC, Bond DJ, Lam RW, Young LT, Yatham LN (2009) Brain-derived neurotrophic factor and inflammatory markers in patients with early- vs. late-stage bipolar disorder. Int J Neuropsychopharmacol 12(4):447-58. Abstract

Kaufman J, Yang BZ, Douglas-Palumberi H, Grasso D, Lipschitz D, Houshyar S, Krystal JH, Gelernter J (2006) Brain-derived neurotrophic factor-5-HTTLPR gene interactions and environmental modifiers of depression in children. Biol Psychiatry 59(8):673-80..

Kaufman J, Yang BZ, Douglas-Palumberi H, Houshyar S, Lipschitz D, Krystal JH, Gelernter J (2004) Social supports and serotonin transporter gene moderate depression in maltreated children. Proc Natl Acad Sci U S A. 101(49):17316-21.

Kempisty B, Bober A, Łuczak M, Czerski P, Szczepankiewicz A, Hauser J, Jagodziński PP (2007) Distribution of 1298A>C polymorphism of methyle-

netetrahydrofolate reductase gene in patients with bipolar disorder and schizophrenia. Eur Psychiatry 22(1):39-43.
Kendler KS, Kuhn JW, Vittum J, Prescott CA, Riley B (2005) The interaction of stressful life events and a serotonin transporter polymorphism in the prediction of episodes of major depression: a replication. Arch Gen Psychiatry 62(5):529-35.
Keikhaee MR, Fadai F, Sargolzaee MR, Javanbakht A, Najmabadi H, Ohadi M (2005) Association analysis of the dopamine transporter (DAT1)-67A/T polymorphism in bipolar disorder.Am J Med Genet B Neuropsychiatr Genet 135B(1):47-9.
Kerner B, Jasinska AJ,DeYoung J, AlmonteM, Choi O-W, Freimer NB (2009) Polymorphisms in the GRIA1 Gene Region in Psychotic Bipolar Disorder. Am J Med Genet Part B 150B:24-32.
Kerner, B, Lambert, CG, Muthen, BO, 2011. Genome-wide association study in bipolar patients stratified by co-morbidity. PLoS One. 6, e28477.
Kessler RC, Berglund P, Demler O, Jin R, Merikangas KR, Walters EE (2005) Lifetime prevalence and age-of-onset distributions of DSM-IV disorders in the National Comorbidity Survey Replication. Arch Gen Psychiatry 62:593-602.
Kieseppä T, Partonen T, Haukka J, Kaprio J, Lönnqvist J (2004) High concordance of bipolar I disorder in a nationwide sample of twins. Am J Psychiatry 161(10):1814-21.
Kim B, Chang Yoon Kim, Hong Pyo Jin, Kim Yoon Seong, Lee Chul (2008) Brain-Derived Neurotrophic Factor Val/Met Polymorphism and Bipolar Disorder. Association with the Met Allele with Suicidal Behaviour of Bipolar Patients. Neuropsychobiology 58:97-103.
Kim HJ, Park HJ, Jung KH, Ban JY, Ra J, Kim JW, Park JK, Choe BK, Yim SV, Kwon YK, Chung JH (2008b) Association study of polymorphisms between DISC1 and schizophrenia in a Korean population. Neurosci Lett 430(1):60-3.
King, DP, Zhao Y, Sangoram, A.M, Wilsbacher LD, Tanaka M, Antoch MP, Steeves TDL, Vitaterna MH, Kornhauser JM, Lowrey PL, Turek FW, Takahashi JS (1997) Positional cloning of the mouse circadian Clock gene. Cell 89: 641-653.
Kishi T, Kitajima T, Ikeda M, Yamanouchi Y, Kinoshita Y, Kawashima K, Okochi T, Okumura T, Tsunoka T, Inada T, Ozaki N, Iwata N (2009) Association study of clock gene (CLOCK) and schizophrenia and mood disorders in the Japanese population. Eur Arch Psychiatry Clin Neurosci 259:293-297
Kirschenbaum B, Goldman SA (1995) Brain-derived neurotrophic factor promotes the survival of neurons arising from the adult rat forebrain subependymal zone. Proc Natl Acad Sci U S A 92(1):210-4

Kirov G, Murphy KC, Arranz MJ, Jones I, McCandles F, Kunugi H, Murray RM, McGuffin P, Collier DA, Owen MJ, Craddock N (1998) Low activity allele of catechol-O-methyltransferase gene associated with rapid cycling bipolar disorder. Mol Psychiatry 3(4):342-5.

Kirov G, Jones I, McCandless F, Craddock N, Owen MJ (1999) Family-based association studies of bipolar disorder with candidate genes involved in dopamine neurotransmission: DBH, DAT1, COMT, DRD2, DRD3 and DRD5. Mol Psychiatry 4(6):558-65

Kirov G, Rees M, Jones I, MacCandless F, Owen MJ, Craddock N (1999) Bipolar disorder and the serotonin transporter gene: a family-based association study. Psychol Med 29(5):1249-54. Abstract

Kishi T, Okochi T, Tsunoka T, Okumura T, Kitajima T, Kawashima K, Yamanouchi Y, Kinoshita Y, Naitoh H, Inada T, Kunugi H, Kato T, Yoshikawa T, Ujike H, Ozaki N, Iwata N.Serotonin 1A receptor gene, schizophrenia and bipolar disorder: an association study and meta-analysis. Psychiatry Res. 2011 Jan 30;185(1-2):20-6. doi: 10.1016/j.psychres.2010.06.003. Epub 2010 Jul 1.

Kishi T, Yoshimura R, Fukuo Y, Okochi T, Matsunaga S, Umene-Nakano W, Nakamura J, Serretti A, Correll CU, Kane JM, Iwata N. The serotonin 1A receptor gene confer susceptibility to mood disorders: results from an extended meta-analysis of patients with major depression and bipolar disorder.Eur Arch Psychiatry Clin Neurosci. 2012 Jul 3.

Klei L, Bacanu SA, Myles-Worsley M, Galke B, Xie W, Tiobech J, Otto C, Roeder K, Devlin B, ByerleyW (2005) Linkage analysis of a completely ascertained sample of familial schizophrenics and bipolars from Palau, Micronesia. Hum Genet 117(4):349-56.

Knippers Rolf (2001) Molekulare Genetik. 8.Auflage.

Kobilka BK., Frielle T, Collins S, Yang-Feng, T, Kobilka T S, Francke U, Lefkowitz RJ, Caron MG (1987) An intronless gene encoding a potential member of the family of receptors coupled to guanine nucleotide regulatory proteins. Nature 329:75-79.

Koenig AM, Thase ME (2009) First-line pharmacotherapies for depression – what is the best choice? Pol Arch Med Wewn 119(7-8):478-86.

Kohen R, Metcalf MA, Khan N, Druck T, Huebner K, Lachowicz JE, Meltzer HY, Sibley DR, Roth BL,Hamblin MW (1996) Cloning, characterization, and chromosomal localization of a human 5-HT6 serotonin receptor. J Neurochem 66(1):47-56.

Kojima H, Ohmori O, Shinkai T, Terao T, Suzuki T, Abe K (1999) Dopamine D1 receptor gene polymorphism and schizophrenia in Japan. Am J Med Genet 88(2):116-9.

Kolupaeva VG, Unbehaun A, Lomakin IB, Hellen CU, Pestova TV (2005) Binding of eukaryotic initiation factor 3 to ribosomal 40S subunits and its role in ribosomal dissociation and anti-association.RNA 11(4):470-86.
Konsensus-Statement – State of the art 2008. Prim. Univ.-Prof. Dr. Michael Bach, Prim. DDr. Christine Butterfield-Meissl,Prim. Univ.-Prof. Dr. Rainer Danzinger, Univ.-Doz. Dr. Andreas Erfurth,Prim. Dr. Ernst-Jörg Friedl, O. Univ.-Prof. Dr. Max Hermann Friedrich,Prim. Univ.-Prof. Dr. Christian Haring, Univ.-Prof. Dr. Armand Hausmann, Dir. Dr. Marion Kalousek, Dr. Claudia Klier, Prim. Univ.-Prof. Dr. Peter König, Prim. Univ.-Prof. DDr. Michael Lehofer, Prim. Dr. Susanne Lentner, Prim. Dr. Thomas Platz, Univ.-Prof. DDr. Gabriele-Maria Sachs, Prim. Univ.-Prof. Dr. Harald Schubert, Prim. Univ.-Prof. Dr. Christian Simhandl, Prim. Univ.-Prof. Dr. Christoph Stuppäck, Prim. Dr. Elmar Windhager,Dr. Wilhelm Wolf, Prim. Dr. Margit Wrobel
Kostrewa D, Zeller ME, Armache KJ, Seizl M, Leike K, Thomm M, Cramer P (2009) RNA polymerase II-TFIIB structure and mechanism of transcription initiation. Nature 462(7271):323-30.
Kostyrko A, Hauser J, Rybakowski JK, Trzeciak WH (2006) Screening of chromosomal region 21q22.3 for mutations in genes associated with neuronal Ca2+ signalling in bipolar affective disorder.Acta Biochim Pol 53(2):317-20.
Krainer AR (1988) Pre-mRNA splicing by complementation with purified human U1,U2, U4/U6 and U5 snRNPs. Nucleic Acids Res 16(20):9415-29.
Krelling R, Cordeiro Q, Miracca E, Gutt EK, Petresco S, Moreno RA, Vallada H (2008) Molecular genetic case-control women investigation from the first Brazilian high-risk study on functional psychosis. Rev Bras Psiquiatr 30(4): 341-5.
Kripke DF, Nievergelt CM, Joo E, Shekhtman T, Kelsoe JR (2009) Circadian polymorphisms associated with affective disorders. Journal of Circadian Rhythms 7:2
Krude T, Jackman M, Pines J, Laskey RA (1997) Cyclin/Cdk-dependent initiation of DNA replication in a human cell-free system. Cell 88(1):109-19.
Krug A, Nieratschker V, Markov V, Krach S, Jansen A, Zerres K, Eggermann T, Stöcker T, Shah NJ, Treutlein J, Mühleisen TW, Kircher T (2010) Effect of CACNA1C rs1006737 on neural correlates of verbal fluency in healthy individuals. Neuroimage 49(2):1831-6.
Kunkel TA, Burgers PM (2008) Dividing the workload at a eukaryotic replication fork. Trends Cell Biol 18(11):521-7.
Kunugi H, Tatsumi M, Sakai T, Hattori M, Nanko S (1996) Serotonin transporter gene polymorphism and affective disorder. Lancet 347(9011):1340.
Kunugi H, Vallada HP, Hoda F, Kirov G, Gill M, Aitchison KJ, Ball D, Arranz MJ, Murray RM, Collier DA (1997) No evidence for an association of affec-

tive disorders with high- or low-activity allele of catechol-omethyltransferase gene. Biol Psychiatry 42(4):282-5.

Kunugi H, Hattori M, Kato T, Tatsumi M, Sakai T, Sasaki T, Hirose T, Nanko S (1997) Serotonin transporter gene polymorphisms: ethnic difference and possible association with bipolar affective disorder. Mol Psychiatry 2(6):457-62.

Kunugi H, Fukuda R, Hattori M, Kato T, Tatsumi M, Sakai T, Hirose T, Nanko S (1998) C677T polymorphism in methylenetetrahydrofolate reductase gene and psychoses. Mol Psychiatry 3(5):435-7.

Kunugi H, Ishida S, Kato T, Tatsumi M, Sakai T, Hattori M, Hirose T and Nanko S (1999) A functional polymorphism in the promoter region of monoamine oxidase-A gene and mood disorders Molecular Psychiatry 4: 393-395

Kunugi H, Iijima Y, Tatsumi M, Yoshida M, Hashimoto R, Kato T, Sakamoto K, Fukunaga T, Inada T, Suzuki T, Iwata N, Ozaki N, Yamada K, Yoshikawa T. No association between the Val66Met polymorphism of the Brain-derived Neurotrophic Factor Gene and Bipolar disorder in a Japanese Population: A Multicenter Study. Biol Psychiatry 2004; 56:376-378

Kvajo M, McKellar H, Arguello PA, Drew LJ, Moore H, MacDermott AB, Karayiorgou M, Gogos JA (2008) A mutation in mouse Disc1 that models a schizophrenia risk allele leads to specific alterations in neuronal architecture and cognition.Proc Natl Acad Sci U S A 105(19):7076-81.

Kwang-Yeon Choi,[1] Ho-Kyoung Yoon,[1] and Yong-Ku Kim Association between Serotonin-Related Polymorphisms in 5HT2A, TPH1, TPH2 Genes and Bipolar Disorder in Korean Population. Psychiatry Investig. 2010 March; 7(1): 60-67.

L:

Lachman HM, Morrow B, Shprintzen R, Veit S, Parsia SS, Faedda G, Goldberg R, Kucherlapati R, Papolos DF (1996) Association of Codon 108/158 Catechol-0-Methyltransferase Gene Polymorphism With the Psychiatric Manifestations of Velo-Cardio-Facial Syndrome. Am J Med Genet 67(5):468-72

Lachman HM, Pedrosa E, Nolan KA, Glass M, Ye K, Saito T (2006) Analysis of polymorphisms in AT-rich domains of neuregulin 1 gene in schizophrenia. Am J Med Genet B Neuropsychiatr Genet 141B(1):102-9

Lachman HM, Stopkova P, Papolos DF, Pedrosa E, Margolis B, Aghalar MR, Saito T (2006) Analysis of synapsin III-196 promoter mutation in schizophrenia and bipolar disorder. Neuropsychobiology 53(2):57-62.

Lachman HM, Pedrosa E, Petruolo OA, Cockerham M, Papolos A, Novak T, Papolos DF, Stopkova P (2007) Increase in GSK3beta gene copy number variation in bipolar disorder. Am J Med Genet B Neuropsychiatr Genet 144B(3):259-65.

Lachman HM (2008) Copy variations in schizophrenia and bipolar disorder. Cytogenet Genome Res 123(1-4):27-35..

Lafuente A, Bernardo M, Mas S, Crescenti A, Aparici M, Gasso P, Deulofeu R, Mane A, Catalan R (2008) Carne X.Polymorphism of dopamine D2 receptor (TaqIA, TaqIB, and-141C Ins/Del) and dopamine degradation enzyme (COMT G158A, A-278G) genes and extrapyramidal symptoms in patients with schizophrenia and bipolar disorders. Psychiatry Res 161(2):131-41.

Lai TJ, Wu CY, Tsai HW, Lin YM, Sun HS (2005) Polymorphism screening and haplotype analysis of the tryptophan hydroxylase gene (TPH1) and association with bipolar affective disorder in Taiwan. BMC Med Genet 6:14.

Langmesser S, Tallone T, Bordon A, Rusconi S, Albrecht U (2008) Interaction of circadian clock proteins PER2 and CRY with BMAL1 and CLOCK. BMC Molecular Biology 2008, 9:41.

Langridge R, Seeds WE, Wilson Hr, Hooper Cw, Wilkins Hf, Hamilton LD (1957) Molecular structure of deoxyribonucleic acid (DNA). J Biophys Biochem Cytol 3(5):767-78.

Lasky-Su JA, Faraone SV, Glatt SJ, Tsuang MT (2005) Meta-analysis of the association between two polymorphisms in the serotonin transporter gene and affective disorders. Am J Med Genet B Neuropsychiatr Genet 133B(1):110-5.

Lee SH, Lee KJ, Lee HJ, Ham BJ, Ryu SH, Lee MS (2005) Association between the 5-HT6 receptor C267T polymorphism and response to antidepressant treatment in major depressive disorder. Psychiatry Clin Neurosci 59(2):140-5.

Lee HC, Tsai SY, Lin HC (2007) Seasonal variations in bipolar disorder admissions and the association with climate: a population-based study. J Affect Disord 97(1-3):61-9

Lee, MT, Chen, CH, Lee, CS, Chen, CC, Chong, MY, Ouyang, WC, Chiu, NY, Chuo, LJ, Chen, CY, Tan, HK, Lane, HY, Chang, TJ, Lin, CH, Jou, SH, Hou, YM, Feng, J, Lai, TJ, Tung, CL, Chen, TJ, Chang, CJ, Lung, FW, Chen, CK, Shiah, IS, Liu, CY, Teng, PR, Chen, KH, Shen, LJ, Cheng, CS, Chang, TP, Li, CF, Chou, CH, Chen, CY, Wang, KH, Fann, CS, Wu, JY, Chen, YT, Cheng, AT, 2011. Genome-wide association study of bipolar I disorder in the Han Chinese population. Mol. Psychiatry. 16, 548-556

Lee SY, Chen SL, Chen SH, Chu CH, Chang YH, Lin SH, Huang SY, Tzeng NS, Kuo PH, Lee IH, Yeh TL, Yang YK, Lu RB.Interaction of the DRD3 and BDNF gene variants in subtyped bipolar disorder. Prog Neuropsychopharmacol Biol Psychiatry. 2012 Dec 3;39(2):382-7. doi: 10.1016/j.pnpbp.2012.07.015. Epub 2012 Jul 31.

Lee SY, Chen SL, Chen SH, Huang SY, Tzeng NS, Chang YH, Wang CL, Lee IH, Yeh TL, Yang YK, Lu RB. World J Biol Psychiatry.The COMT and DRD3 genes interacted in bipolar I but not bipolar II disorder. 2011 Aug;12(5):385-91. doi: 10.3109/15622975.2010.505298. Epub 2010 Aug 10

Lee KY, Joo EJ, Ji YI, Kim DH, Park JB, Chung IW, Lee SI, Joo YH, Ahn YM, Song JY, Kim YS.Associations between DRDs and schizophrenia in a Korean population: multi-stage association analyses. Exp Mol Med. 2011 Jan 31; 43(1):44-52.

Lelli-Chiesa G, Kempton MJ, Jogia J, Tatarelli R, Girardi P, Powell J, Collier DA, Frangou S. The impact of the Val158Met catechol-O-methyltransferase genotype on neural correlates of sad facial affect processing in patients with bipolar disorder and their relatives. Psychol Med. 2011 Apr; 41(4):779-88. doi: 10.1017/S0033291710001431. Epub 2010 Jul 29.

Le-Niculescu H, McFarland MJ, Ogden CA, Balaraman Y, Patel S, Tan J, Rodd ZA, Paulus M, Geyer MA, Edenberg HJ, Glatt SJ, Faraone SV, Nurnberger JI, Kuczenski R, Tsuang MT, Niculescu AB (2008) Phenomic, convergent functional genomic, and biomarker studies in a stress-reactive genetic animal model of bipolar disorder and co-morbid alcoholism. Am J Med Genet B Neuropsychiatr Genet 147B(2):134-66.

Le-Niculescu H, Patel SD, Bhat M, Kuczenski R, Faraone SV, Tsuang MT, McMahon FJ, Schork NJ, Nurnberger JI Jr, Niculescu AB 3rd (2009) Convergent functional genomics of genome-wide association data for bipolar disorder: comprehensive identification of candidate genes, pathways and mechanisms. Am J Med Genet B Neuropsychiatr Genet 150B(2):155-81.

Leszczyńska-Rodziewicz A, Czerski PM, Kapelski P, Godlewski S, Dmitrzak-Weglarz M, Rybakowski J, Hauser J (2002) A polymorphism of the norepinephrine transporter gene in bipolar disorder and schizophrenia: lack of association. Neuropsychobiology 45(4):182-5.

Leszczyńska-Rodziewicz A, Hauser J, Dmitrzak-Weglarz M, Skibińka M, Czerski P, Zakrzewska A, Kosmowska M, Rybakowski JK (2005) Lack of association between polymorphisms of dopamine receptors, type D2, and bipolar affective illness in a Polish population. Med Sci Monit 11(6):CR289-295.

Lemonde S, Turecki G, Bakish D, Du L, Hrdina PD, Bown CD, et al. (2003) Impaired repression at a 5-hydroxytryptamine 1A receptor gene polymorphism associated with major depression and suicide. J Neurosci 23:8788-8799.

Lewis CM, Levinson DF, Wise LH, DeLisi LE, Straub RE, Hovatta I, Williams NM, Schwab SG, Pulver AE, Faraone SV, Brzustowicz LM, Kaufmann CA, Garver DL, Gurling HM, Lindholm E, Coon H, Moises HW, Byerley W, Shaw SH, Mesen A, Sherrington R, O'Neill FA, Walsh D, Kendler KS, Ekelund J, Paunio T, Lönnqvist J, Peltonen L, O'Donovan MC, Owen MJ, Wildenauer DB, Maier W, Nestadt G, Blouin JL, Antonarakis SE, Mowry BJ, Silverman JM, Crowe RR, Cloninger CR, Tsuang MT, Malaspina D, Harkavy-Friedman JM, Svrakic DM, Bassett AS, Holcomb J, Kalsi G, McQuillin A, Brynjolfson J, Sigmundsson T, Petursson H, Jazin E, Zoëga T, Helgason T. (2003) Genome scan meta-analysis of schizophrenia and bipolar disorder, part II: Schizophrenia. Am J Hum Genet 73(1):34-48.

Le-Niculescu H, Patel SD, Bhat M, Kuczenski R, Faraone SV, Tsuang MT, McMahon FJ, Schork NJ, Nurnberger Jr JI, Niculescu III AB (2009) Convergent Functional Genomics of Genome-Wide Association Data for Bipolar Disorder: Comprehensive Identification of Candidate Genes, Pathways and Mechanisms. Am Journal of Medical Genetics Part B 150B:155-181

Lerer B, Macciardi F, Segman RH, Adolfsson R, Blackwood D, Blairy S, Del Favero J, Dikeos DG, Kaneva R, Lilli R, Massat I, Milanova V, Muir W, Noethen M, Oruc L, Petrova T, Papadimitriou GN, Rietschel M, Serretti A, Soucry D, Van Gestel S, Van Broeckhoven C, Mendlewicz J.Variability of 5-HT2C receptor cys23ser polymorphism among European populations and vulnerability to affective disorder. Mol Psychiatry. 2001 Sep;6(5):579-85.

Lewin Benjamin. Genes VIII. 2004.

Li T, Liu X, Sham PC, Aitchison KJ, Cai G, Arranz MJ, Deng H, Liu J, Kirov G, Murray RM, Collier DA (1999) Association analysis between dopamine receptor genes and bipolar affective disorder. Psychiatry Res 86(3):193-201.

Li D, He L (2008) Meta-study on association between the monoamine oxidase A gene (MAOA) and schizophrenia. Am J Med Genet B Neuropsychiatr Genet 147B(2):174-8.

Li X, Zhang J, Wang Y, Ji J, Yang F, Wan C, Wang P, Feng G, Lindpaintner K, He L, He G (2009) Association study on the NAPG gene and bipolar disorder in the Chinese Han population. Neurosci Lett 457(3):159-62.

Li N, He X, Zhang Y, Qi X, Li H, Zhu X, He S.Brain-derived neurotrophic factor signalling mediates antidepressant effects of lamotrigine. Int J Neuropsychopharmacol. 2011 Sep;14(8):1091-8. doi: 10.1017/S1461145710001082. Epub 2010 Sep 16.

Li XW, Liu BC, Wang Y, Zhao QZ, Shen Q, Chen SQ, Ji J, Yang FP, Gao LH, Xu Y, Feng GY, He L, He G. NAPG may not be a common risk gene shared by bipolar disorder and schizophrenia in Chinese population.Psychiatr Genet. 2012 Apr;22(2):107-8. doi: 10.1097/YPG.0b013e32834accd5.

Li Z, Zhang Y, Wang Z, Chen J, Fan J, Guan Y, Zhang C, Yuan C, Hong W, Wang Y, Wu Z, Huang J, Hu Y, Cao L, Yi Z, Cui D, Yu S, Fang Y. The role of BDNF, NTRK2 gene and their interaction in development of treatment-resistant depression: data from multicenter, prospective, longitudinal clinic

practice. J Psychiatr Res. 2013 Jan;47(1):8-14. doi: 10.1016/j.jpsychires. 2012.10.003. Epub 2012 Nov 6.
Lim LCC, Powell JF, Murray R, Gill M (1994) Monoamine oxidase A gene and bipolar affective disorder. (Letter) Am. J. Hum. Genet 54: 1122-1124
Lin YM, Chao SC, Chen TM, Lai TJ, Chen JS, Sun HS (2007) Association of functional polymorphisms of the human tryptophan hydroxylase 2 gene with risk for bipolar disorder in Han Chinese. Arch Gen Psychiatry 64(9):1015-24.
Lin PI, Mitchell BD (2008) Approaches for unraveling the joint genetic determinants of schizophrenia and bipolar disorder. Schizophr Bull 34(4):791-7.
Lin PY (2009) State-dependent decrease in levels of brain-derived neurotrophic factor in bipolar disorder: a meta-analytic study. Neurosci Lett 466(3):139-43.
Liu J, Juo SH, Dewan A, Grunn A, Tong X, Brito M, Park N, Loth JE, Kanyas K, Lerer B, Endicott J, Penchaszadeh G, Knowles JA, Ott J, Gilliam TC, Baron M (2003) Evidence for a putative bipolar disorder locus on 2p13-16 and other potential loci on 4q31, 7q34, 8q13, 9q31, 10q21-24, 13q32, 14q21 and 17q11-12. Mol Psychiatry 8(3):333-42.
Liu, Lixiang, Foroud, Tatiana, Xuei, Xiaoling, Berrettini, Wade, Byerley, William, Coryell, William, El-Mallakh, Rif, Gershon, Elliot, Kelsoe, John, Lawson, William, MacKinnon, Dean, McInnis, Melvin, McMahon, Francis, Murphy, Dennis, Rice, John, Scheftner, William, Zandi, Peter, Lohoff, Falk, Niculescu, Alexander, Meyer, Eric, Edenberg, Howard, Nurnberger, John (2008) Evidence of association between brain-derived neurotrophic factor gene and bipolar disorder. Psychiatric Genetics 18(6):267-274.
Liu ZW, Liu JL, An Y, Zhang L, Wang YM.Association between Ser311Cys polymorphism in the dopamine D2 receptor gene and schizophrenia risk: a meta-analysis in Asian populations. Genet Mol Res. 2012 Feb 8;11(1):261-70. doi: 10.4238/2012.February.8.1.
Lohoff FW, Sander T, Ferraro TN, Dahl JP, Gallinat J and Berrettini WH (2005) Confirmation of Association Between the Val66Met Polymorphism in the Brain-Derived Neurotrophic Factor (BDNF) Gene and Bipolar I Disorder. American Journal of Medical Genetics Part B (Neuropsychiatric Genetics) 139B:51–53.
López-Figueroa AL, Norton CS, López-Figueroa MO, Armellini-Dodel D, Burke S, Akil H, López JF, Watson SJ (2004) Serotonin 5-HT1A, 5-HT1B, and 5-HT2A receptor mRNA expression in subjects with major depression, bipolar disorder, and schizophrenia. Biol Psychiatry 55(3):225-33.
López León S, Croes EA, Sayed-Tabatabaei FA, Claes S, Van Broeckhoven C, van Duijn CM (2005) The dopamine D4 receptor gene 48-base-pair-repeat polymorphism and mood disorders: a meta-analysis.Biol Psychiatry 57(9): 999-1003

López-Muñoz F, Alamo C, Juckel G, Assion HJ (2007) Half a century of antidepressant drugs: on the clinical introduction of monoamine oxidase inhibitors, tricyclics, and tetracyclics. Part I: monoamine oxidase inhibitors. J Clin Psychopharmacol 27(6):555-9.
Lopez VA, Detera-Wadleigh S, Cardona I, National Institute of Mental Health Genetics Initiative Bipolar Disorder Consortium, Kassem L, McMahon FJ (2007) Nested association between genetic variation in tryptophan hydroxylase II, bipolar affective disorder, and suicide attempts. Biol Psychiatry 61(2):181-6.
Lorenzi C, Delmonte D, Pirovano A, Marino E, Bongiorno F, Catalano M, Colombo C, Bramanti P, Smeraldi E (2009) Searching Susceptibility Loci for Bipolar Disorder: A Sib Pair Study on Chromosome 12. Neuropsychobiology 61(1):10-18.
Lorenzi C, Delmonte D, Pirovano A, Marino E, Bongiorno F, Catalano M, Colombo C, Bramanti P, Smeraldi E (2010) Searching susceptibility loci for bipolar disorder: a sib pair study on chromosome 12. Neuropsychobiology 61(1):10-8.
Lorenzo CV, Baca-Garcia E, Hernandez MD, Martin CB, Perez-Rodriguez MM, Saiz Gonzalez MD, Fernández P, Gutierrez FJ, Saiz-Ruiz J, Piqueras JF, de Rivera JL, de Leon J (2007) No association between the Ser9Gly polymorphism of the dopamine D3 receptor gene and schizophrenia in a Spanish sample.Am J Med Genet B Neuropsychiatr Genet 144B(3):344-6.
Lorke DE, Lu G, Cho E, Yew DT (2006) Serotonin 5-HT2A and 5-HT6 receptors in the prefrontal cortex of Alzheimer and normal aging patients. BMC Neurosci 7:36.
Lovejoy EA, Scott AC, Fiskerstrand CE, Bubb VJ, Quinn JP (2003) The serotonin transporter intronic VNTR enhancer correlated with a predisposition to affective disorders has distinct regulatory elements within the domain based on the primary DNA sequence of the repeat unit. Eur J Neurosci 17(2):417-20.
Lucae S, Salyakina D, Barden N, Harvey M, Gagné B, Labbé M, Binder EB, Uhr M, Paez-Pereda M, Sillaber I, Ising M, Brückl T, Lieb R, Holsboer F, Müller-Myhsok B (2006) P2RX7, a gene coding for a purinergic ligand-gated ion channel, is associated with major depressive disorder. Hum Mol Genet 15(16):2438-45.
Lung FW, Tzeng DS, Huang MF, Lee MB.Association of the MAOA promoter uVNTR polymorphism with suicide attempts in patients with major depressive disorder. BMC Med Genet. 2011 May 24;12:74. doi: 10.1186/1471-2350-12-74.

M:

Ma G, He Z, Fang W, Tang W, Huang K, Li Z, He G, Xu Y, Feng G, Zheng T, Zhou J, He L, Shi Y (2008) The Ser9Gly polymorphism of the dopamine D3 receptor gene and risk of schizophrenia: an association study and a large meta-analysis. Schizophr Res 101(1-3):26-35.

MacKenzie A, Quinn J (1999) A serotonin transporter gene intron 2 polymorphic region, correlated with affective disorders, has allele-dependent differential enhancer-like properties in the mouse embryo. Proc Natl Acad Sci U S A 96(26):15251-5.

Maeda K, Nwulia E, Chang J, Balkissoon R, Ishizuka K, Chen H, Zandi P, McInnis MG, Sawa A (2006) Differential expression of disrupted-in-schizophrenia (DISC1) in bipolar disorder. Biol Psychiatry 60(9):929-35.

Maheshwari M, Shi J, Badner JA, Skol A, Willour VL, Muzny DM, Wheeler DA, Gerald FR, Detera-Wadleigh S, McMahon FJ, Potash JB, Gershon ES, Liu C, Gibbs RA (2009) Common and rare variants of DAOA in bipolar disorder.Am J Med Genet B Neuropsychiatr Genet 150B(7):960-6.

Mahieu B, Souery D, Lipp O, Mendelbaum K, Verheyen G, De Maertelaer V, Van Broeckhoven C, Mendlewicz J (1997) No association between bipolar affective disorder and a serotonin receptor (5-HT2A) polymorphism. Psychiatry Res 70(2):65-9.

Mahon PB, Payne JL, MacKinnon DF, Mondimore FM, Goes FS, Schweizer B, Jancic D (2009) NIMH Genetics Initiative Bipolar Disorder Consortium; BiGS Consortium, Coryell WH, Holmans PA, Shi J, Knowles JA, Scheftner WA, Weissman MM, Levinson DF, DePaulo JR Jr, Zandi PP, Potash JB.Genome-wide linkage and follow-up association study of postpartum mood symptoms. Am J Psychiatry 166(11):1229-37.

Maier W (2008) Common risk genes for affective and schizophrenic psychoses. Eur Arch Psychiatry Clin Neurosci 258 Suppl 2:37-40.

Mao Y, Ge X, Frank CL, Madison JM, Koehler AN, Doud MK, Tassa C, Berry EM, Soda T, Singh KK, Biechele T, Petryshen TL, Moon RT, Haggarty SJ, Tsai LH (2009) Disrupted in schizophrenia 1 regulates neuronal progenitor proliferation via modulation of GSK3beta/beta-catenin signaling. Cell 136(6):1017-31.

Meira-Lima I, Michelon L, Cordeiro Q, Cho HJ, Vallada H (2005) Allelic association analysis of the functional insertion/deletion polymorphism in the promoter region of the serotonin transporter gene in bipolar affective disorder. J Mol Neurosci 27(2):219-24.

Malafosse A, Leboyer M, d'Amato T, Amadéo S, Abbar M, Campion D, Canseil O, Castelnau D, Gheysen F, Granger B, Henrikson B, Poirier MF, Sabaté O, Samolyk D, Feingold J, Mallet J (1997) Manic depressive illness and tyrosine

hydroxylase gene: linkage heterogeneity and association. Neurobiol Dis 4(5):337-49.
Mamounas et al. (1995) Brain-derived neurotrophic factor promotes the survival and sprouting of serotonergic axons in rat brain. Journal of Neuroscience 15(12);7929-39
Manchia M, Zai CC, Squassina A, Vincent JB, De Luca V, Kennedy JL. Mixture regression analysis on age at onset in bipolar disorder patients: investigation of the role of serotonergic genes.Eur Neuropsychopharmacol. 2010 Sep; 20(9):663-70. doi: 10.1016/j.euroneuro.2010.04.001. Epub 2010 May 8.
Manchia M, Congiu D, Squassina A, Lampus S, Ardau R, Chillotti C, Severino G, Del Zompo M. No association between lithium full responders and the DRD1, DRD2, DRD3, DAT1, 5-HTTLPR and HTR2A genes in a Sardinian sample. Psychiatry Res. 2009 Sep 30;169(2):164-6. doi: 10.1016/j.psychres. 2008.12.004. Epub 2009 Jul 31.
Manki H, Kanba S, Muramatsu T, Higuchi S, Suzuki E, Matsushita S, Ono Y, Chiba H, Shintani F, Nakamura M, Yagi G, Asai M (1996) Dopamine D2, D3 and D4 receptor and transporter gene polymorphisms and mood disorders. J Affect Disord 40(1-2):7-13.
Mann JJ, Currier D, Murphy L, Huang YY, Galfalvy H, Brent D, Greenhill L, Oquendo M (2008) No association between a TPH2 promoter polymorphism and mood disorders or monoamine turnover. J Affect Disord 106(1-2):117-21.
Mansour HA, Wood J, Logue T, Chowdari KV, Dayal M, Kupfer DJ, Monk TH, Devlin B, Nimgaonkar VL (2006) Association study of eight circadian genes with bipolar I disorder, schizoaffective disorder and schizophrenia.Genes, Brain and Behavior 5: 150-157
Mansour HA, Talkowski ME, Wood J, Chowdari KV, McClain L, Prasad K, Montrose D, Fagiolini A, Friedman ES, Allen MH, Bowden CL, Calabrese J, El-Mallakh RS, Escamilla M, Faraone SV, Fossey MD, Gyulai L, Loftis JM, Hauser P, Ketter TA, Marangell LB, Miklowitz DJ, Nierenberg AA, Patel J, Sachs GS, Sklar P, Smoller JW, Laird N, Keshavan M, Thase ME, Axelson D, Birmaher B, Lewis D, Monk T, Frank E, Kupfer DJ, Devlin B, Nimgaonkar VL(2009) Association study of 21 circadian genes with bipolar I disorder, schizoaffective disorder, and schizophrenia. Bipolar Disord 11(7): 701-10.
Marcheco-Teruel B, Flint TJ, Wikman FP, Torralbas M, González L, Blanco L, Tan Q, Ewald H, Orntoft T, Kruse TA, Børglum AD, Mors O (2006) A genome-wide linkage search for bipolar disorder susceptibility loci in a large and complex pedigree from the eastern part of Cuba. Am J Med Genet B Neuropsychiatr Genet 141B(8):833-43.

Martí SB, Cichon S, Propping P, Nöthen M (2002) Metabotropic glutamate receptor 3 (GRM3) gene variation is not associated with schizophrenia or bipolar affective disorder in the German population. Am J Med Genet 114(1):46-50.

Martinowich K, Lu B (2008) Interaction between BDNF and Serotonin: Role in Mood Disorders. Neuropsychopharmacology 33: 73-83

Martucci L, Wong AH, De Luca V, Likhodi O, Wong GW, King N, Kennedy JL (2006) N-methyl-D-aspartate receptor NR2B subunit gene GRIN2B in schizophrenia and bipolar disorder: Polymorphisms and mRNA levels. Schizophr Res 84(2-3):214-21.

Massat I, Souery D, Del-Favero J, Van Gestel S, Serretti A, Macciardi F, Smeraldi E, Kaneva R, Adolfsson R, Nylander PO, Blackwood D, Muir W, Papadimitriou GN, Dikeos D, Oruc L, Segman RH, Ivezic S, Aschauer H, Ackenheil M, Fuchshuber S, Dam H, Jakovljevic M, Peltonen L, Hilger C, Hentges F, Staner L, Milanova V, Jazin E, Lerer B, Van Broeckhoven C, Mendlewicz J (2002 a) Positive association of dopamine D2 receptor polymorphism with bipolar affective disorder in a European Multicenter Association Study of affective disorders. Am J Med Genet 114(2):177-85.

Massat I, Souery D, Del-Favero J, Oruc L, Noethen MM, Blackwood D, Thomson M, Muir W, Papadimitriou GN, Dikeos DG, Kaneva R, Serretti A, Lilli R, Smeraldi E, Jakovljevic M, Folnegovic V, Rietschel M, Milanova V, Valente F, Van Broeckhoven C, Mendlewicz J (2002 b) Excess of allele1 for alpha3 subunit GABA receptor gene (GABRA3) in bipolar patients: a multicentric association study. Mol Psychiatry 7(2):201-7.

Massat I, Souery D, Del-Favero J, Nothen M, Blackwood D, Muir W, Kaneva R, Serretti A, Lorenzi C, Rietschel M, Milanova V, Papadimitriou GN, Dikeos D, Van Broekhoven C, Mendlewicz J (2005) Association between COMT (Val158Met) functional polymorphism and early onset in patients with major depressive disorder in a European multicenter genetic association study. Mol Psychiatry 10(6):598-605.

Massat I, Kocabas NA, Crisafulli C, Chiesa A, Calati R, Linotte S, Kasper S, Fink M, Antonijevic I, Forray C, Snyder L, Bollen J, Zohar J, De Ronchi D, Souery D, Serretti A, Mendlewicz J.COMT and age at onset in mood disorders: a replication and extension study. Neurosci Lett. 2011 Jul 12;498(3):218-21. doi: 10.1016/j.neulet.2011.05.012. Epub 2011 May 11.

Meyrer R, Demling J, Kornhuber J, Nowak M. Effects of night shifts in bipolar disorders and extreme morningness. Bipolar Disord. 2009 Dec;11(8):897-9. doi: 10.1111/j.1399-5618.2009.00767.

Maziade M, Roy MA, Rouillard E, Bissonnette L, Fournier JP, Roy A, Garneau Y, Montgrain N, Potvin A, Cliche D, Dion C, Wallot H, Fournier A, Nicole L, Lavallée JC, Mérette C (2001) A search for specific and common susceptibility loci for schizophrenia and bipolar disorder: a linkage study in 13 target chromosomes. Mol Psychiatry 6(6):684-93.

Maziade M, Chagnon YC, Roy MA, Bureau A, Fournier A, Mérette C (2009) Chromosome 13q13-q14 locus overlaps mood and psychotic disorders: the relevance for redefining phenotype. Eur J Hum Genet 17(8):1034-42.

McClung CA (2007) Circadian Genes, Rhythms and the Biology of Mood Disorders. Pharmacol Ther 114(2): 222–232.

McGuffin Peter, Rijsdijk Fruhling, Andrew Martin, Sham Pak, Katz Randy, Cardno Alastair (2003) The Heritability of Bipolar Affective Disorder and the Genetic Relationship to Unipolar Depression. Arch Gen Psychiatry 60:497-502

McGuffin P, Knight J, Breen G, Brewster S, Boyd PR, Craddock N, Gill M, Korszun A, Maier W, Middleton L, Mors O, Owen MJ, Perry J, Preisig M, Reich T, Rice J, Rietschel M, Jones L, Sham P, Farmer AE (2005) Whole genome linkage scan of recurrent depressive disorder from the depression network study. Hum Mol Genet 14(22):3337-45.

McInnes LA, Escamilla MA, Service SK, Reus VI, Leon P, Silva S, Rojas E, Spesny M, Baharloo S, Blankenship K, Peterson A, Tyler D, Shimayoshi N, Tobey C, Batki S, Vinogradov S, Meza L, Gallegos A, Fournier E, Smith LB, Barondes SH, Sandkuijl LA, Freimer NB (1996) A complete genome screen for genes predisposing to severe bipolar disorder in two Costa Rican pedigrees. Proc Natl Acad Sci U S A 93(23):13060-5.

McNabb LD, Moore KW, Scena JE, Buono RJ, Berrettini WH (2005) Association analysis of CHMP1.5 genetic variation and bipolar disorder. Psychiatr Genet 15(3):211-4.Abstract

Matute Carlos, Gonzalez-Pinto Ana, Palomino Aitor (2006) Letter to the editor: Decreased levels of plasma BDNF in first-episode schizophrenia and bipolar disorder patients. Schizophrenia Research 86:321-322

Maziade M, Roy MA, Rouillard E, Bissonnette L, Fournier JP, Roy A, Garneau Y, Montgrain N, Potvin A, Cliche D, Dion C, Wallot H, Fournier A, Nicole L, Lavallée JC, Mérette C (2001) A search for specific and common susceptibility loci for schizophrenia and bipolar disorder: a linkage study in 13 target chromosomes. Mol Psychiatry 6(6):684-93.

McAuley EZ, Fullerton JM, Blair IP, Donald JA, Mitchell PB, Schofield PR (2009) Association between the serotonin 2A receptor gene and bipolar affective disorder in an Australian cohort. Psychiatr Genet.19(5):244-52.

Macfadden W, Alphs L, Haskins JT, Turner N, Turkoz I, Bossie C, Kujawa M, Mahmoud R (2009)A randomized, double-blind, placebo-controlled study of maintenance treatment with adjunctive risperidone long-acting therapy in patients with bipolar I disorder who relapse frequently. Bipolar Disord 11(8):827-39.

McDearmon EL, Patel KN, Ko CH, Walisser JA, Schook AC, Chong JL, Wilsbacher LD, Song EJ, Hong HK, Bradfield CA, Takahashi JS (2006) Dissecting the Functions of the Mammalian Clock Protein BMAL1 by Tissue-Specific Rescue in Mice. Science 314(5803):1304-8

McGowan PO, Kato T (2008) Epigenetics in mood disorders.Environ Health Prev Med 13(1):16-24.

McGuffin P, Rijsdijk F, Andrew M, Sham P, Katz R, Cardno A (2003) The heritability of bipolar affective disorder and the genetic relationship to unipolar depression. Arch Gen Psychiatry 60(5):497-502.

McGuffin P, Knight J, Breen G, Brewster S, Boyd PR, Craddock N, Gill M, Korszun A, Maier W, Middleton L, Mors O, Owen MJ, Perry J, Preisig M, Reich T, Rice J, Rietschel M, Jones L, Sham P, Farmer AE (2005) Whole genome linkage scan of recurrent depressive disorder from the depression network study. Hum Mol Genet 14(22):3337-45.

McInnis MG, Dick DM, Willour VL, Avramopoulos D, MacKinnon DF, Simpson SG, Potash JB, Edenberg HJ, Bowman ES, McMahon FJ, Smiley C, Chellis JL, Huo Y, Diggs T, Meyer ET, Miller M, Matteini AT, Rau NL, DePaulo JR, Gershon ES, Badner JA, Rice JP, Goate AM, Detera-Wadleigh SD, Nurnberger JI, Reich T, Zandi PP, Foroud TM (2003) Genome-wide scan and conditional analysis in bipolar disorder: evidence for genomic interaction in the National Institute of Mental Health genetics initiative bipolar pedigrees. Biol Psychiatry 54(11):1265-73.

McInnes LA, Escamilla MA, Service SK, Reus VI, Leon P, Silva S, Rojas E, Spesny M, Baharloo S, Blankenship K, Peterson A, Tyler D, Shimayoshi N, Tobey C, Batki S, Vinogradov S, Meza L, Gallegos A, Fournier E, Smith LB, Barondes SH, Sandkuijl LA, Mendoza J (2006) Circadian Clocks: Setting Time By Food. Journal of Neuroendocrinology 19:127–137

McIntyre RS, Konarski JZ, Jones M, Paulsson B (2007) Quetiapine in the treatment of acute bipolar mania: efficacy across a broad range of symptoms. J Affect Disord 100 Suppl 1:S5-14.

Meira-Lima I, Jardim D, Junqueira R, Ikenaga E, Vallada H.Allelic association study between phospholipase A2 genes and bipolar affective disorder. Bipolar Disord. 2003 Aug;5(4):295-9.

Meloni R, Biguet NF, Mallet J (2002) Post-genomic era and gene discovery for psychiatric diseases: there is a new art of the trade? The example of the HUMTH01 microsatellite in the Tyrosine Hydroxylase gene. Mol Neurobiol 26(2-3):389-403.

Meyer PA, Ye P, Suh MH, Zhang M, Fu J (2009) Structure of the 12-subunit RNA polymerase II refined with the aid of anomalous diffraction data. J Biol Chem 284(19):12933-9.
Mendes de Oliveira JR, Otto PA, Vallada H, Lauriano V, Elkis H, Lafer B, Vasquez L, Gentil V, Passos-Bueno MR, Zatz M (1998) Analysis of a novel functional polymorphism within the promoter region of the serotonin transporter gene (5-HTT) in Brazilian patients affected by bipolar disorder and schizophrenia. Am J Med Genet 81(3):225-7.
Mendlewicz J, Rainer JD (1973) X-linkage in manic-depressive illness. Br Med J 3(5874): 290.
Mendlewicz J, Massat I, Souery D, Del-Favero J, Oruc L, Nöthen MM, Blackwood D, Muir W, Battersby S, Lerer B, Segman RH, Kaneva R, Serretti A, Lilli R, Lorenzi C, Jakovljevic M, Ivezic S, Rietschel M, Milanova V, Van Broeckhoven C (2004) Serotonin transporter 5HTTLPR polymorphism and affective disorders: no evidence of association in a large European multicenter study.Eur J Hum Genet 12(5):377-82.
Mellerup E, Bennike B, Bolwig T, Dam H, Hasholt L, Jørgensen MB, Plenge P, Sørensen SA (2001) Platelet serotonin transporters and the transporter gene in control subjects, unipolar patients and bipolar patients. Acta Psychiatr Scand 103(3):229-33.
Meyer J, Saam W, Mössner R, Cangir Ö, Ortega GR, Tatschner T, Riederer P, Wienker TF, and Lesch KP (2002) Evolutionary conserved microsatellites in the promoter region of the 5-hydroxytryptamine receptor 2C gene (HTR2C) are not associated with bipolar disorder in females. J Neural Transm 109: 939–946
Mick E, Wozniak J, Wilens TE, Biederman J, Faraone SV (2009) Family-based association study of the BDNF, COMT and serotonin transporter genes and DSM-IV bipolar-I disorder in children. BMC Psychiatry 9:2.
Michaud CM, McKenna MT, Begg S, Tomijima N, Majmudar M, Bulzacchelli MT, Ebrahim S, Ezzati M, Salomon JA, Kreiser JG, Hogan M, Murray CJ (1996) The burden of disease and injury in the United States 1996. Popul Health Metr 4:11.
Mill J, Tang T, Kaminsky Z, Khare T, Yazdanpanah S, Bouchard L, Jia P, Assadzadeh A, Flanagan J, Schumacher A, Wang SC, Petronis A (2008) Epigenomic profiling reveals DNA-methylation changes associated with major psychosis.Am J Hum Genet 82(3):696-711.
Millar JK, Wilson-Annan JC, Anderson S, Christie S, Taylor MS, Semple CA, Devon RS, St Clair DM, Muir WJ, Blackwood DH, Porteous DJ (2000) Disruption of two novel genes by a translocation co-segregating with schizophrenia. Hum Mol Genet 9(9):1415-23.

Mino Y, Oshima I, Okagami K (2000) Seasonality of birth in patients with mood disorders in Japan. J Affect Disord 59(1):41-6.

Monteleone P, Serritella C, Martiadis V, Maj M.Decreased levels of serum brain-derived neurotrophic factor in both depressed and euthymic patients with unipolar depression and in euthymic patients with bipolar I and II disorders. Bipolar Disord. 2008 Feb;10(1):95-100.

Moon E, Rollins B, Mesén A, Sequeira A, Myers RM, Akil H, Watson SJ, Barchas J, Jones EG, Schatzberg A, Bunney WE, DeLisi LE, Byerley W, Vawter MP.Lack of association to a NRG1 missense polymorphism in schizophrenia or bipolar disorder in a Costa Rican population. Schizophr Res. 2011 Sep;131(1-3):52-7. doi: 10.1016/j.schres.2011.06.024. Epub 2011 Jul 13.

Moore RY (1999) A clock for the ages.Science 284(5423):2102-3

Moreno FA, Rowe DC, Kaiser B, Chase D, Michaels T, Gelernter J, Delgado PL (2002) Association between a serotonin transporter promoter region polymorphism and mood response during tryptophan depletion. Mol Psychiatry 7(2):213-6.

Morissette J, Villeneuve A, Bordeleau L, Rochette D, Laberge C, Gagné B, Laprise C, Bouchard G, Plante M, Gobeil L, Shink E, Weissenbach J, Barden N (1999) Genome-wide search for linkage of bipolar affective disorders in a very large pedigree derived from a homogeneous population in quebec points to a locus of major effect on chromosome 12q23-q24.Am J Med Genet 88(5):567-87.

Morton NE (1955). "Sequential tests for the detection of linkage". American Journal of Human Genetics **7** (3): 277–318. PMC 1716611. PMID 13258560.

Mühleisen TW, Mattheisen M, Strohmaier J, Degenhardt F, Priebe L, Schultz CC, Breuer R, Meier S, Hoffmann P; GROUP Investigators, Rivandeneira F, Hofman A, Uitterlinden AG, Moebus S, Gieger C, Emeny R, Ladwig KH, Wichmann HE, Schwarz M, Kammerer-Ciernioch J, Schlösser RG, Nenadic I, Sauer H, Mössner R, Maier W, Rujescu D, Lange C, Ophoff RA, Schulze TG, Rietschel M, Nöthen MM, Cichon SAssociation between schizophrenia and common variation in neurocan (NCAN), a genetic risk factor for bipolar disorder. Schizophr Res. 2012 Jun; 138(1):69-73. doi: 10.1016/j.schres.2012.03.007. Epub 2012 Apr 11.

Müller Daniel J, De Luca Vincenzo, Sicard Tricia, King Nicole, Strauss John, Kennedy James (2006) Brain-derived neurotrophic factor (BDNF) gene and rapid cycling disorder. British Yournal of Psychiatry 189:317-323

Müller DJ, Serretti A, Sicard T, Tharmalingam S, King N, Artioli P, Mandelli L, Lorenzi C, Kennedy JL (2007) Further Evidence of MAOAGene Variants Associated With Bipolar Disorder. Am J Med Genet Part B 144:37-40.

Mueller A, Brocke B, Fries E, Lesch KP, Kirschbaum C (2009) The role of the serotonin transporter polymorphism for the endocrine stress response in newborns. Psychoneuroendocrinology. Epub ahead of printing.
Muglia P, Petronis A, Mundo E, Lander S, Cate T, Kennedy JL (2002) Dopamine D4 receptor and tyrosine hydroxylase genes in bipolar disorder: evidence for a role of DRD4.Mol Psychiatry 7(8):860-6.
Mundo E, Zai G, Lee L, Parikh SV, Kennedy JL (2001) The 5HT1Dbeta receptor gene in bipolar disorder: a family-based association study. Neuropsychopharmacology 25(4):608-13.
Mundo E, Walker M, Cate T, Macciardi F, Kennedy JL (2001) The role of serotonin transporter protein gene in antidepressant-induced mania in bipolar disorder: preliminary findings. Arch Gen Psychiatry 58(6):539.
Mundo E, Walker M, Tims H, Macciardi F, Kennedy JL (2000) Lack of linkage disequilibrium between serotonin transporter protein gene (SLC6A4) and bipolar disorder. Am J Med Genet 96(3):379-83.
Muir WJ, Thomson ML, McKeon P, Mynett-Johnson L, Whitton C, Evans KL, Porteous DJ, Blackwood DH (2001) Markers close to the dopamine D5 receptor gene (DRD5) show significant association with schizophrenia but not bipolar disorder.Am J Med Genet 105(2):152-8.
Muramatsu T, Matsushita S, Kanba S, Higuchi S, Manki H, Suzuki E, Asai M (1997) Monoamine oxidase genes polymorphisms and mood disorder. Am J Med Genet 74(5):494-6
Murphy DL, Brodie HK, Goodwin FK, Bunney WE Jr (1971) Regular induction of hypomania by L-dopa in "bipolar" manic-depressive patients. Nature 229(5280):135-6.
Murphy KC, Jones LA, Owen MJ (1999) High rates of schizophrenia in adults with velo-cardio-facial syndrome. Arch Gen Psychiatry 56(10):940-5.
Murphy VE, Mynett-Johnson LA, Claffey E, Bergin P, McAuliffe M, Kealey C, McKeon P (2000) Search for bipolar disorder susceptibility loci: the application of a modified genome scan concentrating on gene-rich regions. Am J Med Genet 96(6):728-32.
Murphy VE, Mynett-Johnson LA, Claffey E, Shields DC, McKeon P (2001) No association between 5HT-2A and bipolar disorder irrespective of genomic imprinting. Am J Med Genet 105(5):422-5.
Murphy DL, Lerner A, Rudnick G, Lesch KP (2004) Serotonin transporter: gene, genetic disorders, and pharmaco-genetics. Mol Interv 4(2):109-23.
Mynett-Johnson L, Kealey C, Claffey E, Curtis D, Bouchier-Hayes L, Powell C, McKeon P (2000) Multimarker-haplotypes within the serotonin transporter gene suggest evidence of an association with bipolar disorder. Am J Med Genet 96(6):845-9.

Miyamoto S, LaMantia AS, Duncan GE, Sullivan P, Gilmore JH, Lieberman JA (2003) Recent advances in the neurobiology of schizophrenia. Mol Interv 3(1):27-39.

N:

Nakata K, Ujike H, Sakai A, Uchida N, Nomura A, Imamura T, Katsu T, Tanaka Y, Hamamura T, Kuroda S (2003) Association study of the brain-derived neurotrophic factor (BDNF) gene with bipolar disorder. Neurosci Lett 337(1):17-20.

Naylor L, Dean B, Pereira A, Mackinnon A, Kouzmenko A, Copolov D (1998) No association between the serotonin transporter-linked promoter region polymorphism and either schizophrenia or density of the serotonin transporter in human hippocampus. Mol Med 4(10):671-4.

Neumeister A, Konstantinidis A, Stastny J, Schwarz MJ, Vitouch O, Willeit M, Praschak-Rieder N, Zach J, de Zwaan M, Bondy B, Ackenheil M, Kasper S (2002) Association between serotonin transporter gene promoter polymorphism (5HTTLPR) and behavioral responses to tryptophan depletion in healthy women with and without family history of depression.Arch Gen Psychiatry 59(7):613-20.

Neves-Pereira M, Mundo E, Muglia P, King N, Macciardi F, Kennedy JL. The Brain-Derived Neurotrophic Factor Gene Confers Susceptibility to Bipolar Disorder: Evidence from a Family-Based Association Study. American journal of human genetics (2002), 71: 651-655

Neves-Pereira M, Cheung JK, Pasdar A, Zhang F, Breen G, Yates P, Sinclair M, Crombie C, Walker N, St Clair DM (2005) BDNF gene is a risk factor for schizophrenia in a Scottish population. Mol Psychiatry 10(2):208-12.

Neves FS, Silveira G, Romano-Silva MA, Malloy-Diniz L, Ferreira AA, De Marco L, Correa H (2008) Is the 5-HTTLPR Polymorphism Associated With Bipolar Disorder or With Suicidal Behavior of Bipolar Disorder Patients? Am J Med Genet Part B 147B:114–116.

Neves FS, Malloy-Diniz LF, Romano-Silva MA, Aguiar GC, de Matos LO, Correa H. Is the serotonin transporter polymorphism (5-HTTLPR) a potential marker for suicidal behavior in bipolar disorder patients? J Affect Disord. 2010 Sep; 125(1-3):98-102. doi: 10.1016/j.jad.2009.12.026. Epub 2010 Jan 21.

Ni X, Trakalo JM, Mundo E, Macciardi FM, Parikh S, Lee L, Kennedy JL (2002) Linkage disequilibrium between dopamine D1 receptor gene (DRD1) and bipolar disorder. Biol Psychiatry 52(12):1144-50.

Nibuya M, Morinobu S, Duman RS. (1995) Regulation of BDNF and trkB mRNA in rat brain by chronic electroconvulsive seizure and antidepressant drug treatments. Journal of Neuroscience 15:7539-7547

Niculescu AB 3rd, Segal DS, Kuczenski R, Barrett T, Hauger RL, Kelsoe JR (2000) Identifying a series of candidate genes for mania and psychosis: a convergent functional genomics approach. Physiol Genomics 4(1):83-91.

Niesler B, Flohr T, Nöthen MM, Fischer C, Rietschel M, Franzek E, Albus M, Propping P, Rappold GA (2001 a) Association between the 5' UTR variant C178T of the serotonin receptor gene HTR3A and bipolar affective disorder. Pharmacogenetics 11(6):471-5. Abstract

Niesler B, Weiss B, Fischer C, Nöthen MM, Propping P, Bondy B, Rietschel M, Maier W, Albus M, Franzek E, Rappold GA (2001 b) Serotonin receptor gene HTR3A variants in schizophrenic and bipolar affective patients. Pharmacogenetics 11(1):21-7. Abstract

Niesler B, Frank B, Kapeller J, Rappold GA (2003) Cloning, physical mapping and expression analysis of the human 5-HT3 serotonin receptor-like genes HTR3C, HTR3D and HTR3E. Gene 310:101-11.

Nielsen DA, Dean M, Goldman D (1992) Genetic mapping of the human tryptophan hydroxylase gene on chromosome 11, using an intronic conformational polymorphism. Am J Hum Genet 51(6):1366-71.

Niesler B, Flohr T, Nöthen MM, Fischer C, Rietschel M, Franzek E, Albus M, Propping P, Rappold GA (2001) Association between the 5' UTR variant C178T of the serotonin receptor gene HTR3A and bipolar affective disorder. Pharmacogenetics 11(6):471-5. Abstract

Niesler B, Kapeller J, Hammer C, Rappold G (2008) Serotonin type 3 receptor genes: HTR3A, B, C, D, E. Pharmacogenomics 9(5):501-4.

Nievergelt CM, Kripke DF, Remick RA, Sadovnick AD, McElroy SL, Keck PE Jr, Kelsoe JR (2005) Examination of the clock gene Cryptochrome 1 in bipolar disorder: mutational analysis and absence of evidence for linkage or association. Psychiatr Genet 15(1):45-52.

Nievergelt CM, Kripke DF, Barrett TB, Burg E, Remick RA, Sadovnick AD, McElroy SL, Keck PE Jr, Schork NJ, Kelsoe JR (2006) Suggestive Evidence for Association of the Circadian Genes PERIOD3 and ARNTL With Bipolar Disorder. American Journal of Medical Genetics Part B (Neuropsychiatric Genetics) 141B:234–241

Nikolov DB, Burley SK (1997) RNA polymerase II transcription initiation: a structural view. Proc Natl Acad Sci U S A 94(1):15-22.

Nonogaki K, Abdallah L, Goulding EH, Bonasera SJ, Tecott LH (2003) Hyperactivity and reduced energy cost of physical activity in serotonin 5-HT(2C) receptor mutant mice. Diabetes 52(2):315-20.

Nöthen MM, Eggermann K, Albus M, Borrmann M, Rietschel M, Körner J, Maier W, Minges J, Lichtermann D, Franzek E, et al. (1995) Association analysis of the monoamine oxidase A gene in bipolar affective disorder by using family-based internal controls.Am J Hum Genet 57(4):975-8.

Nohesara S, Ghadirivasfi M, Mostafavi S, Eskandari MR, Ahmadkhaniha H, Thiagalingam S, Abdolmaleky HM. DNA hypomethylation of MB-COMT promoter in the DNA derived from saliva in schizophrenia and bipolar disorder.J Psychiatr Res. 2011 Nov;45(11):1432-8. doi: 10.1016/j.jpsychires. 2011.06.013. Epub 2011 Aug 5.

Norton N, Kirov G, Zammit S, Jones G, Jones S, Owen R, Krawczak M, Williams NM, O'Donovan MC, Owen MJ (2002) Schizophrenia and functional polymorphisms in the MAOA and COMT genes: no evidence for association or epistasis. Am J Med Genet 114(5):491-6.

Norton N, Williams HJ, Owen MJ (2006) An update on the genetics of schizophrenia. Curr Opin Psychiatry 19:158–164.

Nunokawa A, Watanabe Y, Kaneko N, Sugai T, Yazaki S, Arinami T, Ujike H, Inada T, Iwata N, Kunugi H, Sasaki T, Itokawa M, Ozaki N, Hashimoto R, Someya T (2010) The dopamine D3 receptor (DRD3) gene and risk of schizophrenia: case-control studies and an updated meta-analysis. Schizophr Res 116(1):61-7.

Nyegaard M, Severinsen JE, Als TD, Hedemand A, Straarup S, Nordentoft M, McQuillin A, Bass N, Lawrence J, Thirumalai S, Pereira AC, Kandaswamy R, Lydall GJ, Sklar P, Scolnick E, Purcell S, Curtis D, Gurling HM, Mortensen PB, Mors O, Børglum AD (2009) Support of association between BRD1 and both schizophrenia and bipolar affective disorder. Am J Med Genet B Neuropsychiatr Genet. 2009 Aug 19.

Nyegaard M, Demontis D, Foldager L, Hedemand A, Flint TJ, Sørensen KM, Andersen PS, Nordentoft M, Werge T, Pedersen CB, Hougaard DM, Mortensen PB, Mors O, Børglum AD. CACNA1C (rs1006737) is associated with schizophrenia.Mol Psychiatry. 2010 Feb;15(2):119-21. doi: 10.1038/mp. 2009.69.

O:

Oberlander TF, Weinberg J, Papsdorf M, Grunau R, Misri S, Devlin AM (2008) Prenatal exposure to maternal depression, neonatal methylation of human glucocorticoid receptor gene (NR3C1) and infant cortisol stress responses. Epigenetics 3(2):97-106.

O'Donovan MC, Craddock N, Norton N, Williams H, Peirce T, Moskvina V, Nikolov I, Hamshere M, Carroll L, Georgieva L, Dwyer S, Holmans P, Marchini JL, Spencer CC, Howie B, Leung HT, Hartmann AM, Möller HJ, Morris DW, Shi Y, Feng G, Hoffmann P, Propping P, Vasilescu C, Maier W, Rietschel M, Zammit S, Schumacher J, Quinn EM, Schulze TG, Williams

NM, Giegling I, Iwata N, Ikeda M, Darvasi A, Shifman S, He L, Duan J, Sanders AR, Levinson DF, Gejman PV, Cichon S, Nöthen MM, Gill M, Corvin A, Rujescu D, Kirov G, Owen MJ, Buccola NG, Mowry BJ, Freedman R, Amin F, Black DW, Silverman JM, Byerley WF, Cloninger CR (2008) Molecular Genetics of Schizophrenia Collaboration. Identification of loci associated with schizophrenia by genome-wide association and follow-up. Nat Genet 40(9):1053-5.

Oelgeschläger T, Chiang CM, Roeder RG (1996) Topology and reorganization of a human TFIID-promoter complex. Nature 382(6593):735-8.

Ogilvie AD, Battersby S, Bubb VJ, Fink G, Harmar AJ, Goodwim GM, Smith CA (1996) Polymorphism in serotonin transporter gene associated with susceptibility to major depression. Lancet 347(9003):731-3.

Ohadi M, Keikhaee MR, Javanbakht A, Sargolzaee MR, Robabeh M, Najmabadi H (2007) Gender dimorphism in the DAT1 -67 T-allele homozygosity and predisposition to bipolar disorder. Brain Res 1144:142-5.

Ohara K, Nagai M, Suzuki Y, Ohara K. (1998) Low activity allele of catechol-o-methyltransferase gene and Japanese unipolar depression. Neuroreport. 1998 May 11;9(7):1305-8. Abstract

Ohi K, Hashimoto R, Yasuda Y, Yoshida T, Takahashi H, Iike N, Fukumoto M, Takamura H, Iwase M, Kamino K, Ishii R, Kazui H, Sekiyama R, Kitamura Y, Azechi M, Ikezawa K, Kurimoto R, Kamagata E, Tanimukai H, Tagami S, Morihara T, Ogasawara M, Okochi M, Tokunaga H, Numata S, Ikeda M, Ohnuma T, Ueno S, Fukunaga T, Tanaka T, Kudo T, Arai H, Ohmori T, Iwata N, Ozaki N, Takeda M (2009) Association study of the G72 gene with schizophrenia in a Japanese population: a multicenter study. Schizophr Res 109(1-3):80-5.

Ohlmeier MD, Zhang Y, Bode L, Sieg S, Feutl S, Ludwig H, Emrich HM, Dietrich DE (2008) Amantadine reduces mania in borna disease virus-infected non-psychotic bipolar patients. Pharmacopsychiatry 41(5):202-3.

Ohtsuki T, Ishiguro H, Detera-Wadleigh SD, Toyota T, Shimizu H, Yamada K, Yoshitsugu K, Hattori E, Yoshikawa T, Arinami T (2002) Association between serotonin 4 receptor gene polymorphisms and bipolar disorder in Japanese case-control samples and the NIMH Genetics Initiative bipolar pedigrees. Molec. Psychiat. 7: 954-961.

Oliveira JR, Carvalho DR, Pontual D, Gallindo RM, Sougey EB, Gentil V, Lafer B, Maia LG, Morais MA Jr, Matioli S, Vallada H, Moreno RA, Nishimura A, Otto PA, Passos-Bueno MR, Zatz M (2000) Analysis of the serotonin transporter polymorphism (5-HTTLPR) in Brazilian patients affected by dysthymia, major depression and bipolar disorder. Mol Psychiatry 5(4):348-9.

Ollila HM, Soronen P, Silander K, Palo OM, Kieseppä T, Kaunisto MA, Lönnqvist J, Peltonen L, Partonen T, Paunio T (2009) Findings from bipolar disorder genome-wide association studies replicate in a Finnish bipolar family-cohort. Mol Psychiatry 14(4):351-3.

Okochi T, Ikeda M, Kishi T, Kawashima K, Kinoshita Y, Kitajima T, Yamanouchi Y, Tomita M, Inada T, Ozaki N, Iwata N (2009) Meta-analysis of association between genetic variants in COMT and schizophrenia: an update. Schizophr Res 110(1-3):140-8.

Oruc˘ L , Verheyen GR, Furac I, Jakovljevic M, Ivezic S, Raeymaekers P, and Van Broeckhoven. C (1997 a) Association Analysis of the 5-HT2C Receptor and 5-HT Transporter Genes in Bipolar Disorder. American Journal of Medical Genetics (Neuropsychiatric Genetics) 74:504-506.

Oruc L, Verheyen GR, Furac I, Jakovljević M, Ivezić S, Raeymaekers P, Van Broeckhoven C (1997 b) Analysis of the tyrosine hydroxylase and dopamine D4 receptor genes in a Croatian sample of bipolar I and unipolar patients. Am J Med Genet 74(2):176-8.

Ospina-Duque J, Duque C, Carvajal-Carmona L, Ortiz-Barrientos D, Soto I, Pineda N, Cuartas M, Calle J, Lopez C, Ochoa L, Garcia J, Gomez J, Agudelo A, Lozano M, Montoya G, Ospina A, Lopez M, Gallo A, Miranda A, Serna L, Montoya P, Palacio C, Bedoya G, McCarthy M, Reus V, Freimer N, Ruiz-Linares A (2000) An association study of bipolar mood disorder (type I) with the 5-HTTLPR serotonin transporter polymorphism in a human population isolate from Colombia. Neurosci Lett 292(3):199-202.

Oswald P, Del-Favero J, Massat I, Souery D, Claes S, Van Broeckhoven C, Mendlewicz J (2004)Non Replication in the Brain-Derived Neurotrophic Factor (BDNF) in Bipolar Affective Disorder. A Belgian Patient-Control Study. American Journal of Medical Genetics Part B 129B:24-35

P:

Pae CU, Serretti A, Mandelli L, Yu HS, Patkar AA, Lee CU, Lee SJ, Jun TY, Lee C, Paik IH, Kim JJ (2007) Effect of 5-haplotype of dysbindin gene (DTNBP1) polymorphisms for the susceptibility to bipolar I disorder. Am J Med Genet B Neuropsychiatr Genet 144B(5):701-3.

Pal P, Mihanović M, Molnar S, Xi H, Sun G, Guha S, Jeran N, Tomljenović A, Malnar A, Missoni S, Deka R, Rudan P (2009) Association of tagging single nucleotide polymorphisms on 8 candidate genes in dopaminergic pathway with schizophrenia in Croatian population. Croat Med J 50(4):361-9.

Palo OM, Antila M, Silander K, Hennah W, Kilpinen H, Soronen P, Tuulio-Henriksson A, Kieseppä T, Partonen T, Lönnqvist J, Peltonen L, Paunio T (2007) Association of distinct allelic haplotypes of DISC1 with psychotic and

bipolar spectrum disorders and with underlying cognitive impairments. Hum Mol Genet 16(20):2517-28.
Papadimitriou GN, Dikeos DG, Karadima G, Avramopoulos D, Daskalopoulou EG, Vassilopoulos D, Stefanis CN (1998) Association between the GABA(A) receptor alpha5 subunit gene locus (GABRA5) and bipolar affective disorder.Am J Med Genet 81(1):73-80.
Papadimitriou GN, Dikeos DG, Karadima G, Avramopoulos D, Daskalopoulou EG, Stefanis CN (2001) GABA-A receptor beta3 and alpha5 subunit gene cluster on chromosome 15q11-q13 and bipolar disorder: a genetic association study.Am J Med Genet 105(4):317-20.
Papolos DF, Veit S, Faedda GL, Saito T, Lachman HM (1998) Ultra-ultra rapid cycling bipolar disorder is associated with the low activity catecholamine-O-methyltransferase allele. Mol Psychiatry 3(4):346-9.
Parvin JD, Shykind BM, Meyers RE, Kim J, Sharp PA (1994) Multiple sets of basal factors initiate transcription by RNA polymerase II. J Biol Chem 269(28):18414-21.
Pauls DL, Gerhard DS, Lacy LG, Hostetter AM, Allen CR, Bland SD, LaBuda MC, Egeland JA (1991) Linkage of bipolar affective disorders to markers on chromosome 11p is excluded in a second lateral extension of Amish Pedigree 110. Genomics 11(3) :730-736
Park N, Juo SH, Cheng R, Liu J, Loth JE, Lilliston B, Nee J, Grunn A, Kanyas K, Lerer B, Endicott J, Gilliam TC, Baron M (2004) Linkage analysis of psychosis in bipolar pedigrees suggests novel putative loci for bipolar disorder and shared susceptibility with schizophrenia. Mol Psychiatry 9(12):1091-9.
Parks CL, Robinson PS, Sibille E, Shenk T, Toth M (1998) Increased anxiety of mice lacking the serotonin1A receptor. Proc Natl Acad Sci U S A 95(18): 10734-9.
Parsian A, Todd RD (1997) Genetic Association Between Monoamine Oxidase and Manic-Depressive Illness: Comparison of Relative Risk and Haplotype Relative Risk Data. American Journal of Medical Genetics (Neuropsychiatric Genetics) 74:475–479.
Pearson TA, Manolio TA (2008) How to interpret a genome-wide association study. JAMA 299(11):1335-44.
Peñas-Lledó EM, Dorado P, Cáceres MC, de la Rubia A, Llerena A (2007) Association between T102C and A-1438G polymorphisms in the serotonin receptor 2A (5-HT2A) gene and schizophrenia: relevance for treatment with antipsychotic drugs. Clin Chem Lab Med 45(7):835-8.
PenceaV, Bingaman KD, Wiegand SJ and Luskin MB (2001) Infusion of Brain-Derived Neurotrophic Factor into the Lateral Ventricle of the Adult Rat

Leads to New Neurons in the Parenchyma of the Striatum, Septum, Thalamus, and Hypothalamus. The Journal of Neuroscience 21(17):6706-6717

Pekkarinen P, Terwilliger J, Bredbacka PE, Lönnqvist J, Peltonen L (1995) Evidence of a predisposing locus to bipolar disorder on Xq24-q27.1 in an extended Finnish pedigree. Genome Res 5(2):105-15.

Pereira DS, Tufik S, Louzada FM, Benedito-Silva AA, Lopez AR, Lemos NA, Korczak AL, D'Almeida V, Pedrazzoli M (2005) Association of the length polymorphism in the human Per3 gene with the delayed sleep-phase syndrome: does latitude have an influence upon it? Sleep 28(1):29-32.

Pereira AC, McQuillin A, Puri V, Anjorin A, Bass N, Kandaswamy R, Lawrence J, Curtis D, Sklar P, Purcell SM, Gurling HM. Genetic association and sequencing of the insulin-like growth factor 1 gene in bipolar affective disorder.Am J Med Genet B Neuropsychiatr Genet. 2011 Mar;156(2):177-87. doi: 10.1002/ajmg.b.31153. Epub 2011 Jan 13

Pérez de Castro I, Torres P, Fernández-Piqueras J, Saiz-Ruiz J, Llinares C (1994) No association between dopamine D4 receptor polymorphism and manic depressive illness. J Med Genet 31(11):897-8.

Pérez de Castro I, Santos J, Torres P, Visedo G, Saiz-Ruiz J, Llinares C, Fernández-Piqueras J (1995) A weak association between TH and DRD2 genes and bipolar affective disorder in a Spanish sample. J Med Genet 32(2):131-4.

Perlis RH, Purcell S, Fagerness J, Kirby A, Petryshen TL, Fan J, Sklar P (2008) Family-based association study of lithium-related and other candidate genes in bipolar disorder. Arch Gen Psychiatry 65(1):53-61.

Perlis RH, Smoller JW, Ferreira MA, McQuillin A, Bass N, Lawrence J, Sachs GS, Nimgaonkar V, Scolnick EM, Gurling H, Sklar P, Purcell S (2009) A genomewide association study of response to lithium for prevention of recurrence in bipolar disorder. Am J Psychiatry 166(6):718-25.

Peters UH (2006) Homage to Kraepelin, honouring his 150th birthday – "Zerfahrenheit", Kraepelin's specific symptom for schizophrenia. Fortschr Neurol Psychiatr 74(11):656-64.

Peters JM, Mooney RA, Kuan PF, Rowland JL, Keles S, Landick R (2009) Rho directs widespread termination of intragenic and stable RNA transcription. Proc Natl Acad Sci U S A 106(36):15406-11.

Petryshen TL, Sabeti PC, KA Aldinger, B Fry, JB Fan, SF Schaffner, SG Waggoner, AR Tahl and P Sklar (2006) Population genetic study of the brain derived neurotrophic factor (BDNF) gene. Molecular Psychiatry 1-6

Pezawas L, Verchinski BA, Mattay VS, Callicott JH, Kolachana BS, Straub RE, Egan MF, Meyer-Lindenberg A, Weinberger DR (2004) The brain-derived neurotrophic factor val66met polymorphism and variation in human cortical morphology. J Neurosci 24(45):10099-102.

Psychiatric GWAS Consortium Bipolar Disorder Working Group.Large-scale genome-wide association analysis of bipolar disorder identifies a new susceptibility locus near ODZ4. Nat Genet. 2011 Sep 18;43(10):977-83. doi: 10.1038/ng.943.

Piccardi MP, Severino G, Bocchetta A, Palmas MA, Ruiu S, Del Zompo M (1997) No evidence of association between dopamine D3 receptor gene and bipolar affective disorder. Am J Med Genet 74(2):137-9.

Pickard BS, Malloy MP, Christoforou A, Thomson PA, Evans KL, Morris SW, Hampson M, Porteous DJ, Blackwood DH, Muir WJ. Cytogenetic and genetic evidence supports a role for the kainate-type glutamate receptor gene, GRIK4, in schizophrenia and bipolar disorder. Mol Psychiatry. 2006 Sep;11(9):847-57. Epub 2006 Jul 4.

Pickard BS, Knight HM, Hamilton RS, Soares DC, Walker R, Boyd JK, Machell J, Maclean A, McGhee KA, Condie A, Porteous DJ, St Clair D, Davis I, Blackwood DH, Muir WJ (2008) A common variant in the 3'UTR of the GRIK4 glutamate receptor gene affects transcript abundance and protects against bipolar disorder.Proc Natl Acad Sci U S A 105(39):14940-5.

Pini P (1996) First isolation of Borna disease virus in affective disorder The Lancet 348 (9022): 256

Polanczyk G, Caspi A, Williams B, Price TS, Danese A, Sugden K, Uher R, Poulton R, Moffitt TE (2009) Protective effect of CRHR1 gene variants on the development of adult depression following childhood maltreatment: replication and extension. Arch Gen Psychiatry 66(9):978-85

Poltorak M, Frye MA, Wright R, Hemperly JJ, George MS, Pazzaglia PJ, Jerrels SA, Post RM, Freed WJ (1996) Increased neural cell adhesion molecule in the CSF of patients with mood disorder. J Neurochem 66(4):1532-8.

Pooley EC, Fairburn CG, Cooper Z, Sodhi MS, Cowen PJ, Harrison PJ (2004) A 5-HT2C receptor promoter polymorphism (HTR2C – 759C/T) is associated with obesity in women, and with resistance to weight loss in heterozygotes. Am J Med Genet B Neuropsychiatr Genet 126B(1):124-7.

Porterfield V, Mintz E (2009) Temporal patterns of light-induced immediate-early gene expression in the suprachiasmatic nucleus Neuroscience Letters 463:70-73

Prata DP, Breen G, Osborne S, Munro J, St Clair D, Collier DA (2009) An association study of the neuregulin 1 gene, bipolar affective disorder and psychosis. Psychiatr Genet 19(3):113-6.Abstract

Preisig M, Bellivier F, Fenton BT, Baud P, Berney A, Courtet P, Hardy P, Golaz J, Leboyer M, Mallet J, Matthey ML, Mouthon D, Neidhart E, Nosten-Bertrand M, Stadelmann-Dubuis E, Guimon J, Ferrero F, Buresi C, Malafosse A (2000) Association between bipolar disorder and monoamine oxidase A gene polymorphisms: results of a multicenter study.Am J Psychiatry 157(6):948-55.

Q:

Qiu HT, Meng HQ, Song C, Xiu MH, Chen da C, Zhu FY, Wu GY, Kosten TA, Kosten TR, Zhang XY (2009) Association between monoamine oxidase (MAO)-A gene variants and schizophrenia in a Chinese population. Brain Res 1287:67-73.

R:

Radua J, Surguladze SA, Marshall N, Walshe M, Bramon E, Collier DA, Prata DP, Murray RM, McDonald C.The impact of CACNA1C allelic variation on effective connectivity during emotional processing in bipolar disorder. Mol Psychiatry. 2012 May 22. doi: 10.1038/mp.2012.61.

Ram Murthy A, Purushottam M, Kiran Kumar HB, ValliKiran M, Krishna N, Jayramu Sriharsha K, Janardhan Reddy YC, Ghosh S, Jain S.Gender-specific association of TSNAX/DISC1 locus for schizophrenia and bipolar affective disorder in South Indian population. J Hum Genet. 2012 Aug;57(8):523-30. doi: 10.1038/jhg.2012.62. Epub 2012 Jun 7.

Ramamoorthy S, Bauman AL, Moore KR, Han H, Yang-Feng T, Chang AS, Ganapathy V, Blakely RD (1993) Antidepressant- and cocaine-sensitive human serotonin transporter: molecular cloning, expression, and chromosomal localization. Proc Natl Acad Sci U S A 90(6):2542-6.

Ramboz S, Oosting R, Amara DA, Kung HF, Blier P, Mendelsohn M, Mann JJ, Brunner D, Hen R (1998) Serotonin receptor 1A knockout: an animal model of anxiety-related disorder. Proc Natl Acad Sci U S A 95(24):14476-81.

Raspè E, Mautino G, Duval C, Fontaine C, Duez H, Barbier O, Monte D, Fruchart J, Fruchart JC, Staels B (2002) Transcriptional Regulation of Human Rev-erb Gene Expression by the Orphan Nuclear Receptor Retinoic Acid-related Orphan Receptor. THE JOURNAL OF BIOLOGICAL CHEMISTRY 277 (51):49275-49281.

Raybould R, Green EK, MacGregor S, Gordon-Smith K, Heron J, Hyde S, Caesar S, Nikolov I, Williams N, Jones L, O'Donovan MC, Owen MJ, Jones I, Kirov G, Craddock N (2005) Bipolar disorder and polymorphisms in the dysbindin gene (DTNBP1). Biol Psychiatry 57(7):696-701.

Redon R, Ishikawa S, Fitch KR, Feuk L, Perry GH, Andrews TD, Fiegler H, Shapero MH, Carson AR, Chen W, Cho EK, Dallaire S, Freeman JL, González JR, Gratacòs M, Huang J, Kalaitzopoulos D, Komura D, MacDonald JR, Marshall CR, Mei R, Montgomery L, Nishimura K, Okamura K, Shen F, Somerville MJ, Tchinda J, Valsesia A, Woodwark C, Yang F, Zhang J, Zerjal T, Zhang J, Armengol L, Conrad DF, Estivill X, Tyler-Smith C, Carter NP, Aburatani H, Lee C, Jones KW, Scherer SW, Hurles ME (2006) Global variation in copy number in the human genome. Nature 444(7118):444-54.

Refojo D, Holsboer F (2009) CRH signaling. Molecular specificity for drug targeting in the CNS. Ann N Y Acad Sci 1179:106-19.

Rees S, den Daas I, Foord S, Goodson S, Bull D, Kilpatrick G, Lee M (1994) Cloning and characterisation of the human 5-HT5A serotonin receptor. FEBS Lett 355: 242-246

Rees M, Norton N, Jones I, McCandless F, Scourfield J, Holmans P, Moorhead S, Feldman E, Sadler S, Cole T, Redman K, Farmer A, McGuffin P, Owen MJ, Craddock N (1997) Association studies of bipolar disorder at the human serotonin transporter gene (hSERT; 5HTT). Mol Psychiatry 2(5):398-402.

Remus D, Beuron F, Tolun G, Griffith JD, Morris EP, Diffley JF (2009) Concerted loading of Mcm2-7 double hexamers around DNA during DNA replication origin licensing. Cell 139(4):719-30.

Réthelyi JM, Bakker SC, Polgár P, Czobor P, Strengman E, Pásztor PI, Kahn RS, Bitter I (2009) Association study of NRG1, DTNBP1, RGS4, G72/G30, and PIP5K2A with schizophrenia and symptom severity in a Hungarian sample.Am J Med Genet B Neuropsychiatr Genet. 2009 Nov 24.

Rietschel M, Schorr A, Albus M, Franzek E, Kreiner R, Held T, Knapp M, Müller DJ, Schulze TG, Propping P, Maier W, Nöthen MM (2000) Association study of the tryptophan hydroxylase gene and bipolar affective disorder using family-based internal controls. Am J Med Genet 96(3):310-1.

Rietschel M, Beckmann L, Strohmaier J, Georgi A, Karpushova A, Schirmbeck F, Boesshenz KV, Schmäl C, Bürger C, Jamra RA, Schumacher J, Höfels S, Kumsta R, Entringer S, Krug A, Markov V, Maier W, Propping P, Wüst S, Kircher T, Nöthen MM, Cichon S, Schulze TG (2008) G72 and its association with major depression and neuroticism in large population-based groups from Germany. Am J Psychiatry 165(6):753-62.

Ripperger JA, Shearman LP, Reppert SM, Schibler U (2000) CLOCK, an essential pacemaker component, controls expression of the circadian transcription factor DBP. GENES & DEVELOPMENT 14:679-689.

Robertson E, Jones I, Middle F, Moray J, Craddock N (2003) No association between two polymorphisms at the 5HT2A gene and bipolar affective puerperal psychosis. Acta Psychiatr Scand 108(5):387-91.

Robinson OJ, Sahakian BJ (2009) Acute tryptophan depletion evokes negative mood in healthy females who have previously experienced concurrent negative mood and tryptophan depletion. Psychopharmacology (Berl) 205(2):227-35.

Roche S, McKeon P.Support for tryptophan hydroxylase-2 as a susceptibility gene for bipolar affective disorder. Psychiatr Genet. 2009 Jun;19(3):142-6. doi: 10.1097/YPG.0b013e32832a4f95.

Roeder RG, Lasker Basic (2003) Medical Research Award. The eukaryotic transcriptional machinery: complexities and mechanisms unforeseen. Nat Med 9(10):1239-44.

Rosa A, Cuesta MJ, Fatjó-Vilas M, Peralta V, Zarzuela A, Fañanás L (2006)The Val66Met polymorphism of the brain-derived neurotrophic factor gene is associated with risk for psychosis: Evidence from a family-based association study. Am J Med Genet B Neuropsychiatr Genet 141B(2):135-138.

Rosa A, Picchioni MM, Kalidindi S, Loat CS, Knight J, Toulopoulou T, Vonk R, van der Schot AC, Nolen W, Kahn RS, McGuffin P, Murray RM, Craig IW (2008) Differential methylation of the X-chromosome is a possible source of discordance for bipolar disorder female monozygotic twins. Am J Med Genet B Neuropsychiatr Genet147B(4):459-62.

Rosenthal NE, Mazzanti CM, Barnett RL, Hardin TA, Turner EH, Lam GK, Ozaki N, Goldman D (1998) Role of serotonin transporter promoter repeat length polymorphism (5-HTTLPR) in seasonality and seasonal affective disorder. Mol Psychiatry 3(2):175-7.

Roth BL, Willins DL, Kristiansen K, Kroeze WK (1998) 5-Hydroxytryptamine2-family receptors (5hydroxytryptamine 2A, 5-hydroxytryptamine2B, 5-hydroxytryptamine2C): where structure meets function. Pharmacol Ther 79(3):231-57.

Roy K, Murtie JC, El-Khodor BF, Edgar N, Sardi SP, Hooks BM, Benoit-Marand M, Chen C, Moore H, O'Donnell P, Brunner D, Corfas G (2007) Loss of erbB signaling in oligodendrocytes alters myelin and dopaminergic function, a potential mechanism for neuropsychiatric disorders. Proc Natl Acad Sci U S A.104(19):8131-6.

Roybal K, Theobold D, Graham A, DiNieri JA, Russo SJ, Krishnan V, Chakravarty S, Peevey J, Oehrlein N, Birnbaum S, Vitaterna MH, Orsulak P, Takahashi JS, Nestler EJ, Carlezon WA Jr, McClung CA (2007) Mania-like behavior induced by disruption of CLOCK. Proc Natl Acad Sci U S A.104(15): 6406-11.

Roze E (2008) Pathophysiology of Huntington's disease: from huntingtin functions to potential treatments. Current Opinion in Neurology 21:497–503.

Rothenhäusler HB. Kompendium Praktische Psychiatrie. Springer Verlag. 2007.

Rousseva A, Henry C, van den Bulke D, Fournier G, Laplanche JL, Leboyer M, Bellivier F, Aubry JM, Baud P, Boucherie M, Buresi C, Ferrero F, Malafosse A (2003) Antidepressant-induced mania, rapid cycling and the serotonin transporter gene polymorphism. Pharmacogenomics J 3(2):101-4.

Roussos P, Bitsios P, Giakoumaki SG, McClure MM, Hazlett EA, New AS, Siever LJ. CACNA1C as a risk factor for schizotypal personality disorder

and schizotypy in healthy individuals. Psychiatry Res. 2012 Sep 14. pii: S0165-1781(12)00471-4. doi: 10.1016/j.psychres.2012.08.039.
Rucci P, Nimgaonkar VL, Mansour H, Miniati M, Masala I, Fagiolini A, Cassano GB, Frank E (2009) Gender moderates the relationship between mania spectrum and serotonin transporter polymorphisms in depression. Am J Med Genet B Neuropsychiatr Genet 150B(7):907-13.
Ruiz-Perez VL, Carter SA, Healy E, Todd C, Rees JL, Steijlen PM, Carmichael AJ, Lewis HM, Hohl D, Itin P, Vahlquist A, Gobello T, Mazzanti C, Reggazini R, Nagy G, Munro CS, Strachan T (1999) ATP2A2 mutations in Darier's disease: variant cutaneous phenotypes are associated with missense mutations, but neuropsychiatric features are independent of mutation class.Hum Mol Genet 8(9):1621-30.
Rybakowski JK, Suwalska A, Czerski PM, Dmitrzak-Weglarz M, Leszczynska-Rodziewicz A, Hauser J (2005) Prophylactic effect of lithium in bipolar affective illness may be related to serotonin transporter genotype. Pharmacol Rep 57(1):124-7.
Rybakowski JK, Suwalska A, Skibinska M, Szczepankiewicz A, Leszczynska-Rodziewicz A, Permoda A, Czerski PM, Hauser J (2005) Prophylactic lithium response and polymorphism of the brain-derived neurotrophic factor gene. Pharmacopsychiatry 38(4):166-70.
Rybakowski JK, Suwalska A, Skibinska M, Dmitrzak-Weglarz M, Leszczynska-Rodziewicz A, Hauser J (2007) Response to lithium prophylaxis: interaction between serotonin transporter and BDNF genes. Am J Med Genet B Neuropsychiatr Genet 144B(6):820-3.
Rybakowski JK (2008)BDNF gene: functional Val66Met polymorphism in mood disorders and schizophrenia. Pharmacogenomics 9(11):1589-1593.
Rybakowski JK, Dmitrzak-Weglarz M, Suwalska A, Leszczynska-Rodziewicz A, Hauser J (2009) Dopamine D1 receptor gene polymorphism is associated with prophylactic lithium response in bipolar disorder. Pharmacopsychiatry 42(1):20-2.

S:

Sabol SZ, Hu S, Hamer D (1998) A functional polymorphism in the monoamine oxidase A gene promoter. Hum Genet 103:273-279.
Saito T, Parsia S, Papolos DF, Lachman HM (2000) Analysis of the pseudo-autosomal X-linked gene SYBL1in bipolar affective disorder: description of a new candidate allele for psychiatric disorders. Am J Med Genet 96(3):317-23
Saiyad M, El-Mallakh RS. Smoking is associated with greater symptom load in bipolar disorder patients.Ann Clin Psychiatry. 2012 Nov; 24(4):305-9.

Sáiz PA, García-Portilla MP, Arango C, Morales B, Arias B, Corcoran P, Fernández JM, Alvarez V, Coto E, Bascarán MT, Bousoño M, Fañanas L, Bobes J. Genetic polymorphisms in the dopamine-2 receptor (DRD2), dopamine-3 receptor (DRD3), and dopamine transporter (SLC6A3) genes in schizophrenia: Data from an association study. Prog Neuropsychopharmacol Biol Psychiatry. 2010 Feb 1;34(1):26-31. doi: 10.1016/j.pnpbp.2009.09.008. Epub 2009 Sep 17.

Saleem Q, Ganesh S, Vijaykumar M, Reddy YC, Brahmachari SK, Jain S (2000) Association analysis of 5HT transporter gene in bipolar disorder in the Indian population. Am J Med Genet 96(2):170-2.

Salvatore M, Morzunov S, Schwemmle M, Lipkin WI (1997) Borna disease virus in brains of North American and European people with schizophrenia and bipolar disorder. Bornavirus Study Group. Lancet 349(9068):1813-4.

Sanders SL, Jennings J, Canutescu A, Link AJ, Weil PA (2002) Proteomics of the eukaryotic transcription machinery: identification of proteins associated with components of yeast TFIID by multidimensional mass spectrometry. Mol Cell Biol 22(13):4723-38.

Sanjuan J, Martin-Santos R, Garcia-Esteve L, Carot JM, Guillamat R, Gutierrez-Zotes A, Gornemann I, Canellas F, Baca-Garcia E, Jover M, Navines R, Valles V, Vilella E, de Diego Y, Castro JA, Ivorra JL, Gelabert E, Guitart M, Labad A, Mayoral F, Roca M, Gratacos M, Costas J, van Os J, de Frutos R (2008) Mood changes after delivery: role of the serotonin transporter gene.Br J Psychiatry 193(5):383-8.

Sasaki T, Macciardi FM, Badri F, Verga M, Meltzer HY, Lieberman J, Howard A, Bean G, Joffe RT, Hudson CJ, Kennedy JL (1996) No evidence for association of dopamine D2 receptor variant (Ser311/Cys311) with major psychosis. Am J Med Genet 67(4):415-7.

Savitz J, Lucki I, Drevets WC (2009) 5-HT(1A) receptor function in major depressive disorder. Prog Neurobiol 88(1):17-31.

Savoye C, Laurent C, Amadeo S, Gheysen F, Leboyer M, Lejeune J, Zarifian E, Mallet J (1998) No association between dopamine D1, D2, and D3 receptor genes and manic-depressive illness. Biol Psychiatry 44(7):644-7.

Szczepankiewicz A, Dmitrzak-Weglarz M, Skibínska M, Słopień A, Leszczyńska-Rodziewicz A, Czerski P, Hauser J (2007) Study of dopamine receptors genes polymorphisms in bipolar patients with comorbid alcohol abuse. Alcohol Alcohol 42(2):70-4.

Scholz CJ, Jacob CP, Buttenschon HN, Kittel-Schneider S, Boreatti-Hümmer A, Zimmer M, Walter U, Lesch KP, Mors O, Kneitz S, Deckert J, Reif A (2010) Functional variants of TSPAN8 are associated with bipolar disorder and schizophrenia. Am J Med Genet B Neuropsychiatr Genet.

Schosser A, Gaysina D, Cohen-Woods S, Chow PC, Martucci L, Craddock N, Farmer A, Korszun A, Gunasinghe C, Gray J, Jones L, Tozzi F, Perry J, Muglia P, Owen MJ, Craig IW, McGuffin P (2009) Association of DISC1 and TSNAX genes and affective disorders in the depression case-control (DeCC) and bipolar affective case-control (BACCS) studies. Mol Psychiatry Abstract

Schosser A, Cohen-Woods S, Gaysina D, Chow PC, Martucci L, Farmer A, Korszun A, Gunashinghe C, Gray J, Jones L, Craddock N, Owen MJ, Craig IW, McGuffin P (2010) NRG1 gene in recurrent major depression: No association in a large-scale case-control association study. Am J Med Genet B Neuropsychiatr Genet 153B(1):141-7.

Schosser A, Calati R, Serretti A, Massat I, Kocabas NA, Papageorgiou K, Linotte S, Mendlewicz J, Souery D, Zohar J, Juven-Wetzler A, Montgomery S, Kasper S. The impact of COMT gene polymorphisms on suicidality in treatment resistant major depressive disorder – a European multicenter study. Eur Neuropsychopharmacol. 2012 Apr; 22(4):259-66. doi: 10.1016/j.euroneuro.2011.08.007. Epub 2011 Sep 21.

Schulte-Körne G (2008) Genetik depressiver Störungen. Zeitschrift für Kinder- und Jugendpsychiatrie und Psychotherapie 36:27-43

Schulze TG, Detera-Wadleigh SD, Akula N, Gupta A, Kassem L, Steele J, Pearl J, Strohmaier J, Breuer R, Schwarz M, Propping P, Nöthen MM, Cichon S, Schumacher J (2008) NIMH Genetics Initiative Bipolar Disorder Consortium, Rietschel M, McMahon FJ. Two variants in Ankyrin 3 (ANK3) are independent genetic risk factors for bipolar disorder. Mol Psychiatry 14(5):487-91.

Schulze TG, Alda M, Adli M, Akula N, Ardau R, Bui ET, Chillotti C, Cichon S, Czerski P, Del Zompo M, Detera-Wadleigh SD, Grof P, Gruber O, Hashimoto R, Hauser J, Hoban R, Iwata N, Kassem L, Kato T, Kittel-Schneider S, Kliwicki S, Kelsoe JR, Kusumi I, Laje G, Leckband SG, Manchia M, Macqueen G, Masui T, Ozaki N, Perlis RH, Pfennig A, Piccardi P, Richardson S, Rouleau G, Reif A, Rybakowski JK, Sasse J, Schumacher J, Severino G, Smoller JW, Squassina A, Turecki G, Young LT, Yoshikawa T, Bauer M, McMahon FJ.The International Consortium on Lithium Genetics (ConLiGen): an initiative by the NIMH and IGSLI to study the genetic basis of response to lithium treatment. Neuropsychobiology. 2010;62(1):72-8. doi: 10.1159/000314708. Epub 2010 May 8.

Schumacher J, Jamra RA, Becker T, Ohlraun S, Klopp N, Binder EB, Schulze TG, Deschner M, Schmäl C, Höfels S, Zobel A, Illig T, Propping P, Holsboer F, Rietschel M, Nöthen MM, Cichon S (2005) Evidence for a relationship between genetic variants at the brain-derived neurotrophic factor (BDNF) locus and major depression. Biol Psychiatry 58(4):307-14.

Schumacher J, Kaneva R, Jamra RA, Diaz GO, Ohlraun S, Milanova V, Lee YA, Rivas F, Mayoral F, Fuerst R, Flaquer A, Windemuth C, Gay E, Sanz S, González MJ, Gil S, Cabaleiro F, del Rio F, Perez F, Haro J, Kostov C, Chorbov V, Nikolova-Hill A, Stoyanova V, Onchev G, Kremensky I, Strauch K, Schulze TG, Nürnberg P, Gaebel W, Klimke A, Auburger G, Wienker TF, Kalaydjieva L, Propping P, Cichon S, Jablensky A, Rietschel M, Nöthen MM (2005) Genomewide Scan and Fine-Mapping Linkage Studies in Four European Samples with Bipolar Affective Disorder Suggest a New Susceptibility. Locus on Chromosome 1p35-p36 and Provides Further Evidence of Loci on Chromosome 4q31 and 6q24. Am. J. Hum. Genet 77:1102-1111, 2005

Schumacher J, Laje G, Abou Jamra R, Becker T, Mühleisen TW, Vasilescu C, Mattheisen M, Herms S, Hoffmann P, Hillmer AM, Georgi A, Herold C, Schulze TG, Propping P, Rietschel M, McMahon FJ, Nöthen MM, Cichon S (2009) The DISC locus and schizophrenia: evidence from an association study in a central European sample and from a meta-analysis across different European populations. Hum Mol Genet 18(14):2719-27. Abstract

Schulze TG, Ohlraun S, Czerski PM, Schumacher J, Kassem L, Deschner M, Gross M, Tullius M, Heidmann V, Kovalenko S, Jamra RA, Becker T, Leszczynska-Rodziewicz A, Hauser J, Illig T, Klopp N, Wellek S, Cichon S, Henn FA, McMahon FJ, Maier W, Propping P, Nöthen MM, Rietschel M (2005) Genotype-phenotype studies in bipolar disorder showing association between the DAOA/G30 locus and persecutory delusions: a first step toward a molecular genetic classification of psychiatric phenotypes. Am J Psychiatry 162(11):2101-8.

Schizophrenia Psychiatric Genome-Wide Association Study (GWAS) Consortium.Genome-wide association study identifies five new schizophrenia loci. Nat Genet. 2011 Sep 18;43(10):969-76. doi: 10.1038/ng.940.

Scott LJ, Muglia P, Kong XQ, Guan W, Flickinger M, Upmanyu R, Tozzi F, Li JZ, Burmeister M, Absher D, Thompson RC, Francks C, Meng F, Antoniades A, Southwick AM, Schatzberg AF, Bunney WE, Barchas JD, Jones EG, Day R, Matthews K, McGuffin P, Strauss JS, Kennedy JL, Middleton L, Roses AD, Watson SJ, Vincent JB, Myers RM, Farmer AE, Akil H, Burns DK, Boehnke M (2009) Genome-wide association and meta-analysis of bipolar disorder in individuals of European ancestry. Proc Natl Acad Sci U S A.18: 7501-6.

Sears C, Markie D, Olds R, Fitches A.Evidence of associations between bipolar disorder and the brain-derived neurotrophic factor (BDNF) gene. Bipolar Disord. 2011 Nov-Dec;13(7-8):630-7. doi: 10.1111/j.1399-5618.2011.00955.x.

Segurado R, Detera-Wadleigh SD, Levinson DF, Lewis CM, Gill M, Nurnberger JI Jr, Craddock N, DePaulo JR, Baron M, Gershon ES, Ekholm J, Cichon S,

Turecki G, Claes S, Kelsoe JR, Schofield PR, Badenhop RF, Morissette J, Coon H, Blackwood D, McInnes LA, Foroud T, Edenberg HJ, Reich T, Rice JP, Goate A, McInnis MG, McMahon FJ, Badner JA, Goldin LR, Bennett P, Willour VL, Zandi PP, Liu J, Gilliam C, Juo SH, Berrettini WH, Yoshikawa T, Peltonen L, Lönnqvist J, Nöthen MM, Schumacher J, Windemuth C, Rietschel M, Propping P, Maier W, Alda M, Grof P, Rouleau GA, Del-Favero J, Van Broeckhoven C, Mendlewicz J, Adolfsson R, Spence MA, Luebbert H, Adams LJ, Donald JA, Mitchell PB, Barden N, Shink E, Byerley W, Muir W, Visscher PM, Macgregor S, Gurling H, Kalsi G, McQuillin A, Escamilla MA, Reus VI, Leon P, Freimer NB, Ewald H, Kruse TA, Mors O, Radhakrishna U, Blouin JL, Antonarakis SE, Akarsu N (2003) Genome scan meta-analysis of schizophrenia and bipolar disorder, part III: Bipolar disorder. Am J Hum Genet 73(1):49-62.

Serretti A, Macciardi F, Verga M, Cusin C, Pedrini S, Smeraldi E (1998) Tyrosine hydroxylase gene associated with depressive symptomatology in mood disorder. Am J Med Genet 81(2):127-30.

Serretti A, Macciardi F, Cusin C, Lattuada E, Lilli R, Smeraldi E (1998 b) Dopamine receptor D4 gene is associated with delusional symptomatology in mood disorders. Psychiatry Res 80(2):129-36.

Seretti A, Cusin C, Lattuada E, Di Bella D, Catalano M, Smeraldi E (1999 a) Serotonin transporter gene (5-HTTLPR) is not associated with depressive symptomatology in mood disorders. Mol Psychiatry 4(3):280-3.

Serretti A, Cusin C, Lattuada E, Lilli R, Lorenzi C, Di Bella D, Catalano M, Smeraldi E (1999 b) No interaction between serotonin transporter gene and dopamine receptor D4 gene in symptomatology of major psychoses. Am J Med Genet 88(5):481-5.

Serretti A, Lilli R, Di Bella D, Bertelli S, Nobile M, Novelli E, Catalano M, Smeraldi E (1999 c) Dopamine receptor D4 gene is not associated with major psychoses. Am J Med Genet 88(5):486-91.

Serretti A, Macciardi F, Catalano M, Bellodi L, Smeraldi E (1999 d) Genetic variants of dopamine receptor D4 and psychopathology. Schizophr Bull 25(3):609-18.

Serretti A, Lilli R, Lorenzi C, Lattuada E, Smeraldi E (2000) Serotonin-2C and serotonin-1A receptor genes are not associated with psychotic symptomatology of mood disorders. Am J Med Genet 96(2):161-6.

Serretti A, Macciardi F, Cusin C, Lattuada E, Souery D, Lipp O, Mahieu B, Van Broeckhoven C, Blackwood D, Muir W, Aschauer HN, Heiden AM, Ackenheil M, Fuchshuber S, Raeymaekers P, Verheyen G, Kaneva R, Jablensky A, Papadimitriou GN, Dikeos DG, Stefanis CN, Smeraldi E, Mendlewicz J (2000b)

Linkage of mood disorders with D2, D3 and TH genes: a multicenter study. J Affect Disord 58(1):51-61.
Serretti A, Zanardi R, Rossini D, Cusin C, Lilli R, Smeraldi E (2001) Influence of tryptophan hydroxylase and serotonin transporter genes on fluvoxamine antidepressant activity. Mol Psychiatry 6(5):586-92.
Serretti A, Lilli R, Lorenzi C, Lattuada E, Cusin C, Smeraldi E (2001) Tryptophan hydroxylase gene and major psychoses. Psychiatry Res 103(1):79-86.
Serretti A, Lilli R, Lorenzi C, Lattuada E, Smeraldi E (2001) DRD4 exon 3 variants associated with delusional symptomatology in major psychoses: a study on 2,011 affected subjects. Am J Med Genet 105(3):283-90.
Serretti A, Zanardi R, Rossini D, Cusin C, Lilli R, Smeraldi E (2001b) Influence of tryptophan hydroxylase and serotonin transporter genes on fluvoxamine antidepressant activity. Mol Psychiatry 6(5):586-92.
Serretti A, Cristina S, Lilli R, Cusin C, Lattuada E, Lorenzi C, Corradi B,Grieco G, Costa A, Santorelli F, Barale F, Nappi G, Smeraldi E (2002) Family-based association study of 5-HTTLPR, TPH, MAO-A, and DRD4 polymorphisms in mood disorders. Am J Med Genet 114:361-369.
Serretti A, Malitas PN, Mandelli L, Lorenzi C, Ploia C, Alevizos B, Nikolaou C, Boufidou F, Christodoulou GN, Smeraldi E (2004) Further evidence for a possible association between serotonin transporter gene and lithium prophylaxis in mood disorders. Pharmacogenomics J 4(4):267-73.
Serretti A, Lorenzi C, Mandelli L, Cichon S, Schumacher J, Nöthen MM, Rietschel M, Tullius M, Ohlraun S (2004) DRD4 exon 3 variants are not associated with symptomatology of major psychoses in a German population.Neurosci Lett 368(3):269-73.
Serretti A, Artioli P, Zanardi R, Lorenzi C, Rossini D, Cusin C, Arnoldi A, Catalano M (2004) Genetic features of antidepressant induced mania and hypo-mania in bipolar disorder. Psychopharmacology (Berl) 174(4):504-11.
Serretti A, Cusin C, Rossini D, Artioli P, Dotoli D, Zanardi R (2004) Further evidence of a combined effect of SERTPR and TPH on SSRIs response in mood disorders. Am J Med Genet B Neuropsychiatr Genet 129B(1):36-40.
Serretti A, Mandelli L, Lorenzi C, Landoni S, Calati R, Insacco C, Cloninger CR (2006) Temperament and character in mood disorders: influence of DRD4, SERTPR, TPH and MAO-A polymorphisms. Neuropsychobiology 53(1):9-16.
Serretti A, Mandelli L, Giegling I, Schneider B, Hartmann AM, Schnabel A, Maurer K, Möller HJ, Rujescu D (2007) HTR2C and HTR1A gene variants in German and Italian suicide attempters and completers. Am J Med Genet B Neuropsychiatr Genet 144B(3):291-9.
Serretti A, Chiesa A, Porcelli S, Han C, Patkar AA, Lee SJ, Park MH, Pae CU. Influence of TPH2 variants on diagnosis and response to treatment in patients with

major depression, bipolar disorder and schizophrenia. Genet B Neuropsychiatr Genet 144B(3):291-9. Psychiatry Res. 2011 Aug 30;189(1):26-32. doi: 10.1016/j.psychres.2011.02.001. Epub 2011 Mar 10.

Severino G, Manchia M, Contu P, Squassina A, Lampus S, Ardau R, Chillotti C, Del Zompo M (2009) Association study in a Sardinian sample between bipolar disorder and the nuclear receptor REV-ERBa gene, a critical component of the circadian clock system.Bipolar Disord 11: 215-220.

Severinsen JE, Bjarkam CR, Kiaer-Larsen S, Olsen IM, Nielsen MM, Blechingberg J, Nielsen AL, Holm IE, Foldager L, Young BD, Muir WJ, Blackwood DH, Corydon TJ, Mors O, Børglum AD (2006) Evidence implicating BRD1 with brain development and susceptibility to both schizophrenia and bipolar affective disorder. Mol Psychiatry 11(12):1126-38. Abstract

Shaikh S, Ball D, Craddock N, Castle D, Hunt N, Mant R, Owen M, Collier D, Gill M (1993) The dopamine D3 receptor gene: no association with bipolar affective disorder. J Med Genet 30(4):308-9.

Shearman LP, Sriram S, Weaver DR, Maywood ES, Chaves I, Zheng B, Kume K, Lee CC, van der Horst GTJ, Hastings MH, Reppert SM (2000) Interacting molecular loops in the mammalian circadian clock. Science 288: 1013-1019.

Sher L, Hardin TA, Greenberg BD, Murphy DL, Li Q, Rosenthal NE (1999) Seasonality associated with the serotonin transporter promoter repeat length polymorphism. Am J Psychiatry 156(11):1837. No abstract available. PMID: 10553760

Shi J, Badner JA, Gershon ES, Liu C (2008)Allelic association of G72/G30 with schizophrenia and bipolar disorder: a comprehensive meta-analysis. Schizophr Res 98(1-3):89-97.

Shi J, Badner JA, Gershon ES, Chunyu L, Willour VL, Potash JB (2009) Further evidence for an association of G72/G30 with schizophrenia in Chinese. Schizophr Res 107(2-3):324-6.

Shifman S, Bronstein M, Sternfeld M, Pisanté A, Weizman A, Reznik I, Spivak B, Grisaru N, Karp L, Schiffer R, Kotler M, Strous RD, Swartz-Vanetik M, Knobler HY, Shinar E, Yakir B, Zak NB, Darvasi A (2004) COMT: a common susceptibility gene in bipolar disorder and schizophrenia. Am J Med Genet B Neuropsychiatr Genet 128B(1):61-4.

Shih JC (2004) Cloning, after cloning, knock-out mice, and physiological functions of MAO A and B. Neurotoxicology 25(1-2):21-30.

Shiino Yayoi, Nakajima Satoru, Ozeki Yuji, Isono Takahiro, Yamada Naoto (2003) Mutation screening of the human period 2 gene in bipolar disorder. Neuroscience letters 338:82-84.

Shink E, Morissette J, Villeneuve A, Bordeleau L, Rochette D, Gagné B, Laprise C, Plante M, Barden N (2002) Support for the presence of bipolar disorder susceptibility loci on chromosome 5: heterogeneity in a homogeneous population in Quebec. Prog Neuropsychopharmacol Biol Psychiatry 26(7-8):1273-7.

Shink E, Harvey M, Tremblay M, Gagné B, Belleau P, Raymond C, Labbé M, Dubé MP, Lafrenière RG, Barden N (2005) Analysis of microsatellite markers and single nucleotide polymorphisms in candidate genes for susceptibility to bipolar affective disorder in the chromosome 12Q24.31 region. Am J Med Genet B Neuropsychiatr Genet 135B(1):50-8.

Siridechadilok B, Fraser CS, Hall RJ, Doudna JA, Nogales E (2005) Structural roles for human translation factor eIF3 in initiation of protein synthesis. Science 310(5753):1513-5.

Skibinska M, Hauser J, Czerski PM, Leszczynska-Rodziewicz A, Kosmowska M, Kapelski P, Slopien A, Zakrzewska M, Rybakowski JK. (2004) Association analysis of brain-derived neurotrophic factor (BDNF) gene Val66Met polymorphism in schizophrenia and bipolar affective disorder. World Journal of Biological Psychiatry 5:215-220

Sklar P, Gabriel SB, McInnis MG, Bennett P, Lim YM, Tsan G, Schaffner S, Kirov G, Jones I, Owen M, Craddock N, DePaulo JR, Lander ES (2002) Family-based association study of 76 candidate genes in bipolar disorder: BDNF is a potential risk locus. Molecular Psychiatry 7: 579-593

Sklar P, Pato MT, Kirby A, Petryshen TL, Medeiros H, Carvalho C, Macedo A, Dourado A, Coelho I, Valente J, Soares MJ, Ferreira CP, Lei M, Verner A, Hudson TJ, Morley CP, Kennedy JL, Azevedo MH, Lander E, Daly MJ, Pato CN (2004) Genome-wide scan in Portuguese Island families identifies 5q31-5q35 as a susceptibility locus for schizophrenia and psychosis. Mol Psychiatry 9(2):213-8.

Sklar P, Smoller JW, Fan J, Ferreira MA, Perlis RH, Chambert K, Nimgaonkar VL, McQueen MB, Faraone SV, Kirby A, de Bakker PI, Ogdie MN, Thase ME, Sachs GS, Todd-Brown K, Gabriel SB, Sougnez C, Gates C, Blumenstiel B, Defelice M, Ardlie KG, Franklin J, Muir WJ, McGhee KA, MacIntyre DJ, McLean A, VanBeck M, McQuillin A, Bass NJ, Robinson M, Lawrence J, Anjorin A, Curtis D, Scolnick EM, Daly MJ, Blackwood DH, Gurling HM, Purcell SM (2008) Whole-genome association study of bipolar disorder. Mol Psychiatry 13(6):558-69.

Sklar, P, Ripke, S, Scott, LJ, Andreassen, OA, Cichon, S, Craddock, N, Edenberg, HJ, Nurnberger, JI,Jr, Rietschel, M, Blackwood, D, Corvin, A, Flickinger, M, Guan, W, Mattingsdal, M, McQuillin, A, Kwan, P, Wienker, TF, Daly, M, Dudbridge, F, Holmans, PA, Lin, D, Burmeister, M, Greenwood, TA, Hamshere, ML, Muglia, P, Smith, EN, Zandi, PP, Nievergelt, CM, McKinney, R, Shilling, PD, Schork, NJ, Bloss, CS, Foroud, T, Koller, DL, Gershon, ES, Liu, C, Badner, JA, Scheftner, WA, Lawson, WB, Nwulia, EA, Hipolito,

M, Coryell, W, Rice, J, Byerley, W, McMahon, FJ, Schulze, TG, Berrettini, W, Lohoff, FW, Potash, JB, Mahon, PB, McInnis, MG, Zollner, S, Zhang, P, Craig, DW, Szelinger, S, Barrett, TB, Breuer, R, Meier, S, Strohmaier, J, Witt, SH, Tozzi, F, Farmer, A, McGuffin, P, Strauss, J, Xu, W, Kennedy, JL, Vincent, JB, Matthews, K, Day, R, Ferreira, MA, O'Dushlaine, C, Perlis, R, Raychaudhuri, S, Ruderfer, D, Hyoun, PL, Smoller, JW, Li, J, Absher, D, Thompson, RC, Meng, FG, Schatzberg, AF, Bunney, WE, Barchas, JD, Jones, EG, Watson, SJ, Myers, RM, Akil, H, Boehnke, M, Chambert, K, Moran, J, Scolnick, E, Djurovic, S, Melle, I, Morken, G, Gill, M, Morris, D, Quinn, E, Muhleisen, TW, Degenhardt, FA, Mattheisen, M, Schumacher, J, Maier, W, Steffens, M, Propping, P, Nothen, MM, Anjorin, A, Bass, N, Gurling, H, Kandaswamy, R, Lawrence, J, McGhee, K, McIntosh, A, McLean, AW, Muir, WJ, Pickard, BS, Breen, G, St Clair, D, Caesar, S, Gordon-Smith, K, Jones, L, Fraser, C, Green, EK, Grozeva, D, Jones, IR, Kirov, G, Moskvina, V, Nikolov, I, O'Donovan, MC, Owen, MJ, Collier, DA, Elkin, A, Williamson, R, Young, AH, Ferrier, IN, Stefansson, K, Stefansson, H, Thornorgeirsson, T, Steinberg, S, Gustafsson, O, Bergen, SE, Nimgaonkar, V, Hultman, C, Landen, M, Lichtenstein, P, Sullivan, P, Schalling, M, Osby, U, Backlund, L, Frisen, L, Langstrom, N, Jamain, S, Leboyer, M, Etain, B, Bellivier, F, Petursson, H, Sigur Sson, E, Muller-Mysok, B, Lucae, S, Schwarz, M, Schofield, PR, Martin, N, Montgomery, GW, Lathrop, M, Oskarsson, H, Bauer, M, Wright, A, Mitchell, PB, Hautzinger, M, Reif, A, Kelsoe, JR, Purcell, SM, Psychiatric GWAS Consortium Bipolar Disorder Working Group, 2011. Large-scale genome-wide association analysis of bipolar disorder identifies a new susceptibility locus near ODZ4. Nat. Genet. 43, 977-983.

Smith et al. (1995) Stress alters the expression of brain-derived neurotrophic factor and neurotrophin-3-mRNAs in the hippocampus. Journal of Neuroscience 15:1768-1777

Smith, EN, Bloss, CS, Badner, JA, Barrett, T, Belmonte, PL, Berrettini, W, Byerley, W, Coryell, W, Craig, D, Edenberg, HJ, Eskin, E, Foroud, T, Gershon, E, Greenwood, TA, Hipolito, M, Koller, DL, Lawson, WB, Liu, C, Lohoff, F, McInnis, MG, McMahon, FJ, Mirel, DB, Murray, SS, Nievergelt, C, Nurnberger, J, Nwulia, EA, Paschall, J, Potash, JB, Rice, J, Schulze, TG, Scheftner, W, Panganiban, C, Zaitlen, N, Zandi, PP, Zollner, S, Schork, NJ, Kelsoe, JR, 2009. Genome-wide association study of bipolar disorder in European American and African American individuals. Mol. Psychiatry. 14, 755-763.

Smith, EN, Koller, DL, Panganiban, C, Szelinger, S, Zhang, P, Badner, JA, Barrett, TB, Berrettini, WH, Bloss, CS, Byerley, W, Coryell, W, Edenberg, HJ, Foroud, T, Gershon, ES, Greenwood, TA, Guo, Y, Hipolito, M, Keating, BJ,

Lawson, WB, Liu, C, Mahon, PB, McInnis, MG, McMahon, FJ, McKinney, R, Murray, SS, Nievergelt, CM, Nurnberger, JI,Jr, Nwulia, EA, Potash, JB, Rice, J, Schulze, TG, Scheftner, WA, Shilling, PD, Zandi, PP, Zollner, S, Craig, DW, Schork, NJ, Kelsoe, JR, 2011. Genome-wide association of bipolar disorder suggests an enrichment of replicable associations in regions near genes. PLoS Genet. 7, e1002134.

Smyth C, Kalsi G, Curtis D, Brynjolfsson J, O'Neill J, Rifkin L, Moloney E, Murphy P, Petursson H, Gurling H (1997) Two-locus admixture linkage analysis of bipolar and unipolar affective disorder supports the presence of susceptibility loci on chromosomes 11p15 and 21q22. Genomics 39(3):271-8.

Soria V, Martínez-Amorós E, Escaramís G, Valero J, Pérez-Egea R, García C, Gutiérrez-Zotes A, Puigdemont D, Bayés M, Crespo JM, Martorell L, Vilella E, Labad A, Vallejo J, Pérez V, Menchón JM, Estivill X, Gratacòs M, Urretavizcaya M. Differential association of circadian genes with mood disorders: CRY1 and NPAS2 are associated with unipolar major depression and CLOCK and VIP with bipolar disorder.Neuropsychopharmacology. 2010 May; 35(6):1279-89. doi: 10.1038/npp.2009.230. Epub 2010 Jan 13.

Soronen P, Mantere O, Melartin T, Suominen K, Vuorilehto M, Rytsälä H, Arvilommi P, Holma I, Holma M, Jylhä P, Valtonen HM, Haukka J, Isometsä E, Paunio T.P2RX7 gene is associated consistently with mood disorders and predicts clinical outcome in three clinical cohorts.Am J Med Genet B Neuropsychiatr Genet. 2011 Jun;156B(4):435-47. doi: 10.1002/ajmg.b.31179. Epub 2011 Mar 22.

Souery D, Lipp O, Mahieu B, Mendelbaum K, De Martelaer V, Van Broeckhoven C, Mendlewicz J (1996) Association study of bipolar disorder with candidate genes involved in catecholamine neurotransmission: DRD2, DRD3, DAT1, and TH genes. Am J Med Genet 67(6):551-5.

Souery D, Lipp O, Rivelli SK, Massat I, Serretti A, Cavallini C, Ackenheil M, Adolfsson R, Aschauer H, Blackwood D, Dam H, Dikeos D, Fuchshuber S, Heiden M, Jakovljevic M, Kaneva R, Kessing L, Lerer B, Lönnqvist J, Mellerup T, Milanova V, Muir W, Nylander PO, Oruc L, Mendlewicz J, et al. (1999) Tyrosine hydroxylase polymorphism and phenotypic heterogeneity in bipolar affective disorder: a multicenter association study. Am J Med Genet 88(5):527-32.

Souery D, Van Gestel S, Massat I, Blairy S, Adolfsson R, Blackwood D, Del-Favero J, Dikeos D, Jakovljevic M, Kaneva R, Lattuada E, Lerer B, Lilli R, Milanova V, Muir W, Nöthen M, Oruc L, Papadimitriou G, Propping P, Schulze T, Serretti A, Shapira B, Smeraldi E, Stefanis C, Thomson M, Van Broeckhoven C, Mendlewicz J (2001) Tryptophan hydroxylase polymorphism and suicidality in unipolar and bipolar affective disorders: a multicenter association study. Biol Psychiatry 49(5):405-9

Squassina A, Manchia M, Manconi F, Piccardi M, Ardau R, Chillotti C, Severino G, Del Zompo M.A case-control association study of the PDLIM5 gene and bipolar disorder in a Sardinian sample. Psychiatr Genet. 2008 Jun;18(3):128-32. doi: 10.1097/YPG.0b013e3282fb003d.

Squassina A, Manchia M, Costa M, Chillotti C, Ardau R, Del Zompo M, Severino G. Age at onset in bipolar disorder: Investigation of the role of TaqIA polymorphism of DRD2 gene in a Sardinian sample.Eur Psychiatry. 2011 Apr;26(3):141-3. Epub 2011 Feb 2.

Stine OC, McMahon FJ, Chen L, Xu J, Meyers DA, MacKinnon DF, Simpson S, McInnis MG, Rice JP, Goate A, Reich T, Edenberg HJ, Foroud T, Nurnberger JI Jr, Detera-Wadleigh SD, Goldin LR, Guroff J, Gershon ES, Blehar MC, DePaulo JR (1997) Initial genome screen for bipolar disorder in the NIMH genetics initiative pedigrees: chromosomes 2, 11, 13, 14, and X. Am J Med Genet 74(3):263-9.

Stöber G, Heils A, Lesch KP (1996) Serotonin transporter gene polymorphism and affective disorder. Lancet 347(9011):1340-1.

Stöber G, Nöthen MM, Pörzgen P, Brüss M, Bönisch H, Knapp M, Beckmann H, Propping P (1996) Systematic search for variation in the human norepinephrine transporter gene: identification of five naturally occurring missense mutations and study of association with major psychiatric disorders. Am J Med Genet 67(6):523-32.

Stratakis CA, Sarlis NJ, Berrettini WH, Badner JA, Chrousos GP, Gershon ES, Detera-Wadleigh SD (1997) Lack of linkage between the corticotropin-releasing hormone (CRH) gene and bipolar affective disorder. Mol Psychiatry 2(6):483-5.

Szczepankiewicz A, Skibinska M, Rybakowski J, Leszczynska-Rodziewicz A, Tomaszewska M, Twarowska-Hauser J (2009) Lack of association of three GRIN2B polymorphisms with bipolar disorder. World J Biol Psychiatry 10:469-73. Abstract

Strauss J, Barr CL, George CJ, King N, Shaikh S, Devlin B, Kovacs M, Kennedy JL (2004) Association study of brain-derived neurotrophic factor in adults with a history of childhood onset mood disorder. Am j med genet neuropsychiatr genet 131B(1);16-9

Sugawara H, Iwamoto K, Bundo M, Ueda J, Miyauchi T, Komori A, Kazuno A, Adati N, Kusumi I, Okazaki Y, Ishigooka J, Kojima T, Kato T. Hypermethylation of serotonin transporter gene in bipolar disorder detected by epigenome analysis of discordant monozygotic twins. Transl Psychiatry. 2011 Jul 26; 1:e24. doi: 10.1038/tp.2011.26.

Sullivan GM, Ogden RT, Oquendo MA, Kumar JS, Simpson N, Huang YY, Mann JJ, Parsey RV (2009) Positron emission tomography quantification of serotonin-1A receptor binding in medication-free bipolar depression.Biol Psychiatry 66(3):223-30.

Suzuki T, Iwata N, Kitamura Y, Kitajima T, Yamanouchi Y, Ikeda M, Nishiyama T, Kamatani N, Ozaki N (2003) Association of a haplotype in the serotonin 5-HT4 receptor gene (HTR4) with Japanese schizophrenia. Am J Med Genet B Neuropsychiatr Genet 121B(1):7-13.

Syagailo YV, Stober G, Grassle M, Reimer E, Knapp M, Jungkunz G, Okladnova O, Meyer J, Lesch KP (2001) Association analysis of the functional monoamine oxidase A gene promoter polymorphism in psychiatric disorders. Am J Med Genet 105:168–171.

Sylvia LG, Ametrano RM, Nierenberg AA (2009) Exercise Treatment for Bipolar Disorder: Potential Mechanisms of Action Mediated through Increased Neurogenesis and Decreased Allostatic Load. Psychother Psychosom 79(2):87-96.

T:

Takata A, Kawasaki H, Iwayama Y, Yamada K, Gotoh L, Mitsuyasu H, Miura T, Kato T, Yoshikawa T, Kanba S.Nominal association between a polymorphism in DGKH and bipolar disorder detected in a meta-analysis of East Asian case-control samples. Psychiatry Clin Neurosci. 2011 Apr;65(3):280-5. doi: 10.1111/j.1440-1819.2011.02193.x.

Talkowski ME, Mansour H, Chowdari KV, Wood J, Butler A, Varma PG, Prasad S, Semwal P, Bhatia T, Deshpande S, Devlin B, Thelma BK, Nimgaonkar VL (2006) Novel, replicated associations between dopamine D3 receptor gene polymorphisms and schizophrenia in two independent samples. Biol Psychiatry 60(6):570-7.

Tarn WY, Steitz JA (1997) Pre-mRNA splicing: the discovery of a new spliceosome doubles the challenge. Trends Biochem Sci 22(4):132-7.

Tecott LH, Sun LM, Akana SF, Strack AM, Lowenstein DH, Dallman MF, Julius D (1995) Eating disorder and epilepsy in mice lacking 5-HT2c serotonin receptors. Nature 374(6522):542-6.

Terayama H, Nishino Y, Kishi M, Ikuta K, Itoh M, Iwahashi K (2003) Detection of anti-Borna Disease Virus (BDV) antibodies from patients with schizophrenia and mood disorders in Japan. Psychiatry Res 120(2):201-6.

Tesli M, Kähler AK, Andreassen BK, Werge T, Mors O, Mellerup E, Koefoed P, Melle I, Morken G, Wirgenes KV, Andreassen OA, Djurovic S. No association between DGKH and bipolar disorder in a Scandinavian case-control sample.Psychiatr Genet. 2009 Oct;19(5):269-72. doi: 10.1097/YPG.0b013e32832d302f.

The Wellcome Trust Case Control ConsortiumGenome-wide association study of 14,000 cases of seven common diseases and 3,000 shared controls (2007) Nature 447(7145): 661-678.

Thomson PA, Wray NR, Millar JK, Evans KL, Hellard SL, Condie A, Muir WJ, Blackwood DH, Porteous DJ (2005) Association between the TRAX/DISC locus and both bipolar disorder and schizophrenia in the Scottish population. Mol Psychiatry 10(7):657-68, 616.

Thomson PA, Macintyre DJ, Hamilton G, Dominiczak A, Smith BH, Morris A, Evans KL, Porteous DJ.Association of DISC1 variants with age of onset in a population-based sample of recurrent major depression. Mol Psychiatry. 2012 Aug. 7. doi: 10.1038/mp.2012.117. [Epub ahead of print]

Tölle R (2008) Eugen Bleuler (1857-1939) and German psychiatry.Nervenarzt 79(1):90-6, 98.

Toh KL, Jones CR, He Y, Eide EJ, Hinz WA, Virshup DM, Ptácek LJ, Fu YH (2001) An hPer2 Phosphorylation Site Mutation in Familial Advanced Sleep Phase Syndrome 291(5506):1040-3.

Tohen M, Vieta E (2009) Antipsychotic agents in the treatment of bipolar mania. Bipolar Disord 2:45-54.

Tomàs C, Cañellas F, Rodríguez V, Picornell A, Lafau O, Nadal M, Roca M, Serrano MJ, Castro JA, Ramon MM (2006) Genetic linkage study for bipolar disorders on chromosomes 17 and 18 in families with a high expression of mental illness from the Balearic Islands. Psychiatr Genet16(4):145-51. Abstract

Tomppo L, Hennah W, Lahermo P, Loukola A, Tuulio-Henriksson A, Suvisaari J, Partonen T, Ekelund J, Lönnqvist J, Peltonen L (2009) Association between genes of Disrupted in schizophrenia 1 (DISC1) interactors and schizophrenia supports the role of the DISC1 pathway in the etiology of major mental illnesses. Biol Psychiatry 65(12):1055-62.

Torrey EF, Rawlings RR, Ennis JM, Merrill DD, Flores DS (1996) Birth seasonality in bipolar disorder, schizophrenia, schizoaffective disorder and stillbirths. Schizophr Res 21(3):141-9.

Tramontina JF, Andreazza AC, Kauer-Sant'anna M, Stertz L, Goi J, Chiarani F, Kapczinski F (2009) Brain-derived neurotrophic factor serum levels before and after treatment for acute mania. Neurosci Lett 452(2):111-3.

Tsai SJ, Chiu HJ, Wang YC, Hong CJ (1999) Association study of serotonin-6 receptor variant (C267T) with schizophrenia and aggressive behavior. Neurosci Lett 271(2):135-7.

Tsai SJ, Hong CJ, Hsu CC, Cheng CY, Liao WY, Song HL, Lai HC (1999) Serotonin-2A receptor polymorphism (102T/C) in mood disorders. Psychiatry Res 87(2-3):233-7.

Tsai SJ, Hong CJ, Wang YC (1999) Tryptophan hydroxylase gene polymorphism (A218C) and suicidal behaviors. Neuroreport 10(18):3773-5.

Tseng M, Alda M, Xu L, Sun X, Wang JF, Grof P, Turecki G, Rouleau G, Young LT (2008) BDNF protein levels are decreased in transformed lymphoblasts from lithium-responsive patients with bipolar disorder. J Psychiatry Neurosci 33(5):449-53.

Tut TG, Wang JL, Lim CC (2000) Negative association between T102C polymorphism at the 5-HT2A receptor gene and bipolar affective disorders in Singaporean Chinese. J Affect Disord 58(3):211-4.

Tyrka AR, Price LH, Gelernter J, Schepker C, Anderson GM, Carpenter LL (2009) Interaction of childhood maltreatment with the corticotropin-releasing hormone receptor gene: effects on hypothalamic-pituitary-adrenal axis reactivity. Biol Psychiatry 66(7):681-5.

U:

Utsunomiya K, Shinkai T, De Luca V, Hwang R, Sakata S, Fukunaka Y, Chen HI, Ohmori O, Nakamura J (2008) Neurosci Lett. 2008 Oct 24;444(2):161-5. Epub 2008 Aug 7.Genetic association between the dopamine D3 gene polymorphism (Ser9Gly) and schizophrenia in Japanese populations: evidence from a case-control study and meta-analysis. Neurosci Lett 444(2):161-5.

V:

Van Den Bogaert A, Sleegers K, De Zutter S, Heyrman L, Norrback KF, Adolfsson R, Van Broeckhoven C, Del-Favero J. Association of brain-specific tryptophan hydroxylase, TPH2, with unipolar and bipolar disorder in a Northern Swedish, isolated population.Arch Gen Psychiatry. 2006 Oct;63(10):1103-10.

Van Tol HH, Bunzow JR, Guan HC, Sunahara RK, Seeman P, Niznik HB, Civelli O (1991) Cloning of the gene for a human dopamine D4 receptor with high affinity for the antipsychotic clozapine.Nature 350(6319):610-4.

Van Tol HH, Wu CM, Guan HC, Ohara K, Bunzow JR, Civelli O, Kennedy J, Seeman P, Niznik HB, Jovanovic V (1992) Multiple dopamine D4 receptor variants in the human population. Nature 358(6382):149-52.

Van Duijn E, Kingma EM, van der Mast RC (2007) Psychopathology in Verified Huntington's Disease Gene Carriers. The Journal of Neuropsychiatry and Clinical Neurosciences 19:441-448

Verma R, Mukerji M, Grover D, B-Rao C (2005) Das SK, Kubendran S, Jain S, Brahmachari SK. MLC1 gene is associated with schizophrenia and bipolar disorder in Southern India. Biol Psychiatry 58(1):16-22.

Videtic A, Zupanc T, Pregelj P, Balazic J, Tomori M, Komel R (2009) Suicide, stress and serotonin receptor 1A promoter polymorphism -1019C>G in Slovenian suicide victims. Eur Arch Psychiatry Clin Neurosci.259(4):234-8.

Videtic A, Peternelj TT, Zupanc T, Balazic J, Komel R (2009) Promoter and functional polymorphisms of HTR2C and suicide victims. Genes Brain Behav 8(5):541-5.

Vincent JB, Masellis M, Lawrence J, Choi V, Gurling HM, Parikh SV, Kennedy JL (1999) Genetic association analysis of serotonin system genes in bipolar affective disorder. Am J Psychiatry. Am J Psychiatry 156(1):136-8.

Vincze I, Perroud N, Buresi C, Baud P. Bellivier F, Etain B, Fournier C, Karege F, Matthey M-L, Preisig M, Leboyer M, Malafosse A (2008) Association between brain-derived neurotrophic factor gene and a severe form of bipolar disorder, but no interaction with the serotonin transporter gene. Bipolar disorders 10: 580-587

Voineskos D, De Luca V, Macgregor S, Likhodi O, Miller L, Voineskos AN, Kennedy JL (2009) Neuregulin 1 and age of onset in the major psychoses. J Neural Transm 116(4):479-86.

Voisey J, Swagell CD, Hughes IP, Lawford BR, Young RM, Morris CP.A novel DRD2 single-nucleotide polymorphism associated with schizophrenia predicts age of onset: HapMap tag-single-nucleotide polymorphism analysis. Genet Test Mol Biomarkers. 2012 Feb;16(2):77-81. doi: 10.1089/gtmb.2011.0085. Epub 2011 Aug 23.

Volpe FM, Del Porto JA (2006) Seasonality of admissions for mania in a psychiatric hospital of Belo Horizonte, Brazil. J Affect Disord 94(1-3):243-8.

Volpe FM, Tavares A, Del Porto JA (2008) Seasonality of three dimensions of mania: psychosis, aggression and suicidality. J Affect Disord 108(1-2):95-100.

Volpe FM, da Silva EM, Dos Santos TN, de Freitas DE (2009) Further evidence of seasonality of mania in the tropics. J Affect Disord. 2009 Nov 19.

W:

Waldman ID, Robinson BF, Feigon SA (1997) Linkage disequilibrium between the dopamine transporter gene (DAT1) and bipolar disorder: extending the transmission disequilibrium test (TDT) to examine genetic heterogeneity. Genet Epidemiol 14(6):699-704.

Walker RM, Christoforou A, Thomson PA, McGhee KA, Maclean A, Mühleisen TW, Strohmaier J, Nieratschker V, Nöthen MM, Rietschel M, Cichon S, Morris SW, Jilani O, Stclair D, Blackwood DH, Muir WJ, Porteous DJ, Evans KL.Association analysis of Neuregulin 1 candidate regions in schizophrenia and bipolar disorder. Neurosci Lett. 2010 Jun 30;478(1):9-13. doi: 10.1016/j.neulet.2010.04.056. Epub 2010 May 7.

Walss-Bass C, Raventos H, Montero AP, Armas R, Dassori A, Contreras S, Liu W, Medina R, Levinson DF, Pereira M, Leach RJ, Almasy L, Escamilla MA (2006) Association analyses of the neuregulin 1 gene with schizophrenia and manic psychosis in a Hispanic population. Acta Psychiatr Scand 113(4):314-21.

Walther DJ, Peter JU, Bashammakh S, Hörtnagl H, Voits M, Fink H, Bader M (2003) Synthesis of serotonin by a second tryptophan hydroxylase isoform. Science 299(5603):76.

Wang Y, Hu Y, Fang Y, Zhang K, Yang H, Ma J, Xu Q, Shen Y (2009) Evidence of epistasis between the catechol-O-methyltransferase and aldehyde dehydrogenase 3B1 genes in paranoid schizophrenia. Biol Psychiatry 65(12):1048-54.

Wang F, McIntosh AM, He Y, Gelernter J, Blumberg HP.The association of genetic variation in CACNA1C with structure and function of a frontotemporal system. Bipolar Disord. 2011 Nov-Dec;13(7-8):696-700. doi: 10.1111/j.1399-5618.2011.00963.x.

Wang Y, Liu X, Yu Y, Han Y, Wei J, Collier D, Li T, Ma X.The role of single nucleotide polymorphism of D(2) dopamine receptor gene on major depressive disorder and response to antidepressant treatment. Psychiatry Res. 2012 Dec 30;200(2-3):1047-50. doi: 10.1016/j.psychres.2012.06.024. Epub 2012 Jul 15.

Wang Z, Li Z, Chen J, Huang J, Yuan C, Hong W, Yu S, Fang Y. Association of BDNF gene polymorphism with bipolar disorders in Han Chinese population.Genes Brain Behav. 2012 Jul;11(5):524-8. doi: 10.1111/j.1601-183X.2012.00797.x. Epub 2012 May 4.

Wasserman D, Geijer T, Sokolowski M, Rozanov V, Wasserman J (2006) The serotonin 1A receptor C(-1019)G polymorphism in relation to suicide attempt. Behav Brain Funct 2

Watanabe Y, Nunokawa A, Kaneko N, Someya T (2007) Meta-analysis of case-control association studies between the C270T polymorphism of the brain-derived neurotrophic factor gene and schizophrenia. Schizophr Res 95(1-3):250-2.

Watson JD, Crick FH (1974) Molecular structure of nucleic acids: a structure for deoxyribose nucleic acid. JD Watson and FHC Crick. Published in Nature, number 4356 April 25, 1953. Nature 248(5451):765.

Watson S, Gallagher P, Ritchie JC, Ferrier IN, Young AH (2004) Hypothalamic-pituitary-adrenal axis function in patients with bipolar disorder. Br J Psychiatry 184:496-502.

Weber H, Kittel-Schneider S, Gessner A, Domschke K, Neuner M, Jacob CP, Buttenschon HN, Boreatti-Hümmer A, Volkert J, Herterich S, Baune BT, Gross-Lesch S, Kopf J, Kreiker S, Nguyen TT, Weissflog L, Arolt V, Mors O, Deckert J, Lesch KP, Reif A. Cross-disorder analysis of bipolar risk genes:

further evidence of DGKH as a risk gene for bipolar disorder, but also unipolar depression and adult ADHD. Neuropsychopharmacology. 2011 Sep; 36(10):2076-85. doi: 10.1038/npp.2011.98. Epub 2011 Jun 8.

Weller AE, Dahl JP, Lohoff FW, Ferraro TN, Berrettini WH (2006) Analysis of variations in the NAPG gene on chromosome 18p11 in bipolar disorder. Psychiatr Genet 16(1):3-8. Abstract

Wessman J, Paunio T, Tuulio-Henriksson A, Koivisto M, Partonen T, Suvisaari J, Turunen JA, Wedenoja J, Hennah W, Pietiläinen OP, Lönnqvist J, Mannila H, Peltonen L (2009) Mixture model clustering of phenotype features reveals evidence for association of DTNBP1 to a specific subtype of schizophrenia. Biol Psychiatry 66(11):990-6.

Wigg K, Feng Y, Gomez L, Kiss E, Kapornai K, Tamás Z, Mayer L, Baji I, Daróczi G, Benák I, Osváth VK, Dombovári E, Kaczvinszk E, Besnyõ M, Gádoros J, King N, Székely J, Kovacs M, Vetró A, Kennedy JL, Barr CL (2009) Genome scan in sibling pairs with juvenile-onset mood disorders: Evidence for linkage to 13q and Xq. Am J Med Genet B Neuropsychiatr Genet 150B(5):638-46.

Wilson GM, Flibotte S, Chopra V, Melnyk BL, Honer WG, Holt RA (2006) DNA copy-number analysis in bipolar disorder and schizophrenia reveals aberrations in genes involved in glutamate signaling. Hum Mol Genet 15(5):743-9.

Wilkie MJ, Smith G, Day RK, Matthews K, Smith D, Blackwood D, Reid IC, Wolf CR (2009) Polymorphisms in the SLC6A4 and HTR2A genes influence treatment outcome following antidepressant therapy. Pharmacogenomics J 9(1):61-70.

Willeit M, Praschak-Rieder N, Neumeister A, Zill P, Leisch F, Stastny J, Hilger E, Thierry N, Konstantinidis A, Winkler D, Fuchs K, Sieghart W, Aschauer H, Ackenheil M, Bondy B, Kasper S (2003) A polymorphism (5-HTTLPR) in the serotonin transporter promoter gene is associated with DSM-IV depression subtypes in seasonal affective disorder.Mol Psychiatry 8(11):942-6.

Willeit M, Sitte HH, Thierry N, Michalek K, Praschak-Rieder N, Zill P, Winkler D, Brannath W, Fischer MB, Bondy B, Kasper S, Singer EA (2008) Enhanced serotonin transporter function during depression in seasonal affective disorder.Neuropsychopharmacology 33(7):1503-13.

Wirgenes KV, Djurovic S, Agartz I, Jonsson EG, Werge T, Melle I, Andreassen OA (2009) Dysbindin and d-amino-acid-oxidase gene polymorphisms associated with positive and negative symptoms in schizophrenia. Neuropsychobiology 60(1):31-6.

Wiste AK, Arango V, Ellis SP, Mann JJ, Underwood MD (2008) Norepinephrine and serotonin imbalance in the locus coeruleus in bipolar disorder. Bipolar Disord 10(3):349-59.

Wray NR, James MR, Dumenil T, Handoko HY, Lind PA, Montgomery GW, Martin NG (2008) Association study of candidate variants of COMT with neuroticism, anxiety and depression. Am J Med Genet B Neuropsychiatr Genet147B(7):1314-8.

Wu SY, Chiang CM (2001) TATA-binding protein-associated factors enhance the recruitment of RNA polymerase II by transcriptional activators.J Biol Chem 276(36):34235-43.

Wu Y, Xu Y, Sun Y, Wang YF, Li X, Lang XE, Wang WP, Zhang KR (2008) Association between the serotonin 1A receptor C(-1019)G polymorphism and major depressive disorder in the northern Han ethnic group in China. Chin Med J (Engl) 121(10):874-6. Abstract

X:

Xiang L, Szebeni K, Szebeni A, Klimek V, Stockmeier CA, Karolewicz B, Kalbfleisch J, Ordway GA (2008) Dopamine receptor gene expression in human amygdaloid nuclei: elevated D4 receptor mRNA in major depression. Brain Res 1207:214-24.

Xiao Y, Zhang J, Wang Y, Wang P, Li X, Ji J, Yang F, Feng G, He L, He G.Limited association between Disrupted in Schizophrenia 1(DISC1) gene and bipolar disorder in the Chinese population.Psychiatr Genet. 2011 Feb; 21(1):42-6.

Xu C, Li PP, Cooke RG, Parikh SV, Wang K, Kennedy JL, Warsh JJ (2009) TRPM2 variants and bipolar disorder risk: confirmation in a family-based association study. Bipolar Disord 11(1):1-10.

Xu J, Liu Y, Wang P, Li S, Wang Y, Li J, Zhou D, Chen Z, Zhao T, Wang T, Xu H, Yang Y, Feng G, He L, Yu L.Positive association between the brain-derived neurotrophic factor (BDNF) gene and bipolar disorder in the Han Chinese population. Am J Med Genet B Neuropsychiatr Genet. 2010 Jan 5; 153B(1):275-9.

Y:

Yamada K, Hattori E, Iwayama Y, Ohnishi T, Ohba H, Toyota T, Takao H, Minabe Y, Nakatani N, Higuchi T, Detera-Wadleigh SD, Yoshikawa T (2006) Distinguishable haplotype blocks in the HTR3A and HTR3B region in the Japanese reveal evidence of association of HTR3B with female major depression. Biol Psychiatry 60(2):192-201.

Yang MQ, Elnitski LL (2008) Diversity of core promoter elements comprising human bidirectional promoters.BMC Genomics 16:9
Yang SA.Association between a Missense Polymorphism (rs3924999, Arg253Gln) of Neuregulin 1 and Schizophrenia in Korean Population. Exp Neurobiol. 2012 Dec; 21(4):158-63. doi: 10.5607/en.2012.21.4.158. Epub 2012 Dec 26.
Yarden G, Elfakess R, Gazit K, Dikstein R (2009) Characterization of sINR, a strict version of the Initiator core promoter element. Nucleic Acids Res 37(13):4234-46.
Yen FC, Hong CJ, Hou SJ, Wang JK, Tsai SJ (2003) Association study of serotonin transporter gene VNTR polymorphism and mood disorders, onset age and suicide attempts in a Chinese sample. Neuropsychobiology 48(1):5-9.
Yin Lei, Wang Jing, Klein Peter S., Lazar Mitchell A (2006) Nuclear Receptor Rev-erba Is a Critical Lithium-Sensitive Component of the Circadian Clock. SCIENCE Vol 311
Yosifova A, Mushiroda T, Stoianov D, Vazharova R, Dimova I, Karachanak S, Zaharieva I, Milanova V, Madjirova N, Gerdjikov I, Tolev T, Velkova S, Kirov G, Owen MJ, O'Donovan MC, Toncheva D, Nakamura Y (2009) Case-control association study of 65 candidate genes revealed a possible association of a SNP of HTR5A to be a factor susceptible to bipolar disease in Bulgarian population. J Affect Disord 117(1-2):87-97.
Yosifova, A, Mushiroda, T, Kubo, M, Takahashi, A, Kamatani, Y, Kamatani, N, Stoianov, D, Vazharova, R, Karachanak, S, Zaharieva, I, Dimova, I, Hadjidekova, S, Milanova, V, Madjirova, N, Gerdjikov, I, Tolev, T, Poryazova, N, O'Donovan, MC, Owen, MJ, Kirov, G, Toncheva, D, Nakamura, Y, 2011. Genome-wide association study on bipolar disorder in the Bulgarian population. Genes Brain Behav. 10, 789-797.
Yu YW, Tsai SJ, Hong CJ, Chen TJ, Chen MC, Yang CW (2005) Association study of a monoamine oxidase a gene promoter polymorphism with major depressive disorder and antidepressant response.Neuropsychopharmacology 30(9):1719-23.
Yu YW, Tsai SJ, Liou YJ, Hong CJ, Chen TJ (2006) Association study of two serotonin 1A receptor gene polymorphisms and fluoxetine treatment response in Chinese major depressive disorders. Eur Neuro-psychopharmacol 16(7):498-503.
Yuan A, Yi Z, Wang Q, Sun J, Li Z, Du Y, Zhang C, Yu T, Fan J, Li H, Yu S. ANK3 as a risk gene for schizophrenia: new data in Han Chinese and meta analysis.Am J Med Genet B Neuropsychiatr Genet. 2012 Dec;159B(8):997-1005. doi: 10.1002/ajmg.b.32112. Epub 2012 Oct 25.

Z:

Zaboli G, Jönsson EG, Gizatullin R, Asberg M, Leopardi R (2006) Tryptophan hydroxylase-1 gene variants associated with schizophrenia. Biol Psychiatry 60(6):563-9.

Zandi PP, Willour VL, Huo Y, Chellis J, Potash JB, MacKinnon DF, Simpson SG, McMahon FJ, Gershon E, Reich T, Foroud T, Nurnberger J Jr, DePaulo JR Jr, McInnis MG; National Institute of Mental Health Genetics Initiative Bipolar Group (2003) Genome scan of a second wave of NIMH genetics initiative bipolar pedigrees: chromosomes 2, 11, 13, 14, and X. Am J Med Genet B Neuropsychiatr Genet 119B(1):69-76

Zandi PP, Belmonte PL, Willour VL, Goes FS, Badner JA, Simpson SG, Gershon ES, McMahon FJ, DePaulo JR Jr, Potash JB; Bipolar Disorder Phenome Group; National Institute of Mental Health Genetics Initiative Bipolar Disorder Consortium (2008) Association study of Wnt signaling pathway genes in bipolar disorder.Arch Gen Psychiatry 65(7):785-93.

Zeng Z, Wang T, Li T, Li Y, Chen P, Zhao Q, Liu J, Li J, Feng G, He L, Shi Y. Common SNPs and haplotypes in DGKH are associated with bipolar disorder and schizophrenia in the Chinese Han population.Mol Psychiatry. 2011 May;16(5):473-5. doi: 10.1038/mp.2010.86. Epub 2010 Aug 24. No abstract available.

Zhang Z, Lindpaintner K, Che R, He Z, Wang P, Yang P, Feng G, He L, Shi Y (2009) The Val/Met functional polymorphism in COMT confers susceptibility to bipolar disorder: evidence from an association study and a meta-analysis. J Neural Transm 116:1193–1200

Zhang D, Cheng L, Qian Y, Alliey-Rodriguez N, Kelsoe JR, Greenwood T, Nievergelt C, Barrett TB, McKinney R, Schork N, Smith EN, Bloss C, Nurnberger J, Edenberg HJ, Foroud T, Sheftner W, Lawson WB, Nwulia EA, Hipolito M, Coryell W, Rice J, Byerley W, McMahon F, Schulze TG, Berrettini W, Potash JB, Belmonte PL, Zandi PP, McInnis MG, Zöllner S, Craig D, Szelinger S, Koller D, Christian SL, Liu C, Gershon ES (2009) Singleton deletions throughout the genome increase risk of bipolar disorder. Mol Psychiatry 14(4):376-80.

Zhang HY, Ishigaki T, Tani K, Chen K, Shih JC, Miyasato K, Ohara K, Ohara K. (1997) Serotonin2A receptor gene polymorphism in mood disorders. Biol Psychiatry 41(7):768-73.

Zhang K, Xu Q, Xu Y, Yang H, Luo J, Sun Y, Sun N, Wang S, Shen Y (2009) The combined effects of the 5-HTTLPR and 5-HTR1A genes modulates the relationship between negative life events and major depressive disorder in a Chinese population. J Affect Disord 114(1-3):224-31.

Zhang JX, Chen YB, Zhang KR, Xu Q, Shen Y.[Association between monoamine oxidase A gene and major depression in Chinese Han population]. Zhongguo Yi Xue Ke Xue Yuan Xue Bao. 2009 Dec;31(6):728-34. doi: 10.3881/j.issn.1000-503X.2009.06.015

Zhang Q, Shen Q, Xu Z, Chen M, Cheng L, Zhai J, Gu H, Bao X, Chen X, Wang K, Deng X, Ji F, Liu C, Li J, Dong Q, Chen C.The effects of CACNA1C gene polymorphism on spatial working memory in both healthy controls and patients with schizophrenia or bipolar disorder. Neuropsychopharmacology. 2012 Feb;37(3):677-84. doi: 10.1038/npp.2011.242. Epub 2011 Oct 19.

Zhao T, Liu Y, Wang P, Li S, Zhou D, Zhang D, Chen Z, Wang T, Xu H, Feng G, He L, Yu L (2009) Positive association between the PDLIM5 gene and bipolar disorder in the Chinese Han population.J Psychiatry Neurosci. 34(3): 199-204

Zhao C, Xu Z, Wang F, Chen J, Ng SK, Wong PW, Yu Z, Pun FW, Ren L, Lo WS, Tsang SY, Xue H (2009) Alternative-splicing in the exon-10 region of GABA(A) receptor beta(2) subunit gene: relationships between novel isoforms and psychotic disorders. PLoS One 4(9)

Zheng C, Shen Y, Xu Q.Rs1076560, a functional variant of the dopamine D2 receptor gene, confers risk of schizophrenia in Han Chinese. Neurosci Lett. 2012 Jun 14;518(1):41-4. doi: 10.1016/j.neulet.2012.04.052. Epub 2012 Apr 30.

Zhou X, Barrett TB, Kelsoe JR (2008) Promoter variant in the GRK3 gene associated with bipolar disorder alters gene expression.Biol Psychiatry 64(2):104-10.

Zigova T, Pencea V, Wiegand SJ, Luskin MB (1998) Intraventricular Administration of BDNF Increases the Number of Newly Generated Neurons in the Adult Olfactory Bulb Molecular and Cellular Neuroscience 11 (4): 234-245

Zill P, Baghai TC, Engel R, Zwanzger P, Schüle C, Eser D, Behrens S, Rupprecht R, Möller HJ, Ackenheil M, Bondy B (2004) The dysbindin gene in major depression: an association study. Am J Med Genet B Neuropsychiatr Genet 129B(1):55-8.

Zou F, Li C, Duan S, Zheng Y, Gu N, Feng G, Xing Y, Shi J, He L (2005) A family-based study of the association between the G72/G30 genes and schizophrenia in the Chinese population.Schizophr Res 73(2-3):257-61.

Zou YF, Wang F, Feng XL, Li WF, Tian YH, Tao JH, Pan FM, Huang F. Association of DRD2 gene polymorphisms with mood disorders: a meta-analysis. J Affect Disord. 2012 Feb;136(3):229-37. Epub 2010 Dec 4.

Zhu F, Yan CX, Wang Q, Zhu YS, Zhao Y, Huang J, Zhang HB, Gao CG, Li SB. An association study between dopamine D1 receptor gene polymorphisms and the risk of schizophrenia. Brain Res. 2011 Oct 28;1420:106-13. doi: 10.1016/j.brainres.2011.08.069. Epub 2011 Sep 5.

Zubenko GS, Maher B, Hughes HB 3rd, Zubenko WN, Stiffler JS, Kaplan BB, Marazita ML (2003) Genome-wide linkage survey for genetic loci that influence the development of depressive disorders in families with recurrent, early-onset, major depression. Am J Med Genet B Neuropsychiatr Genet 123B(1):1-18.

www.ingramcontent.com/pod-product-compliance
Ingram Content Group UK Ltd.
Pitfield, Milton Keynes, MK11 3LW, UK
UKHW021832100926
8556IPUK00004B/293

9 783631 635728